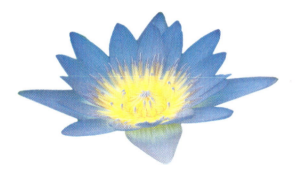

CURE YOURSELF WITH
YOGA

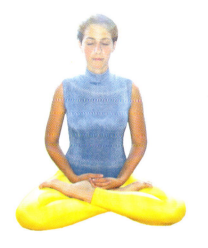

Ácárya Hiranmayánanda Avt.

Cure Yourself With Yoga
Dádá Ác. Hirańmayánanda Avt.

1st Edition - May 2004
2nd Edition - Dec 2006
Copyright reserved to the author and to the publisher

ISBN : 975-92052 -1-1

The author of this book does not dispense medical advise nor prescribes the use of any technique as a form of treatment for medical problems without the advise of a physician who knows yoga techniques or a competent yoga teacher, either directly or indirectly.

No part of this book maybe produced or used by any mechanical, photographic, or electronic process, or in the form of a phonographic recording, nor may it be stored in a retrieval system, transmitted, or otherwise copied for public or private use without the written permission of the publisher.

Kozmik Dans ve Yayıncılık Ltd
Hamam Sokak 84/2 Caddebostan / İstanbul - TURKEY
Telephone: 90 216 369 84 68 - 302 01 14
E-mail: kipyoga@yahoo.com

Design and colour fixing by
Mavi Renk Ayrım

Printed & Published in India by
Vision Creative Services
108, JE-9, Khirki Ext. Malviya Nagar, New Delhi - 17

Dedication

This work is offered to my most Beloved Master,
Shrii Shrii Ánandamúrti
That personality who means everything to my
life.
While preparing this book, I was merely the
instrument.
The hands that wrote it were mine, but the real
writer is He.
What more can I say than,
"Oh my beloved JAGAT GURU, all Your treasures,
I offer back to You"

Hiranmayánanda

CONTENTS

INDEX FOR THE DISEASES	4
PREFACE	6
INTRODUCTION	8
HISTORY	12
YOGA PHILOSOPHY	16
CAKRAS AND KOŚAS	18
AŚTÁUNGA YOGA AND KOŚA	23
CAKRAS	24
THE EIGHT STEPS OF SELF-REALISATION	
AŚTÁUNGA YOGA	30
YOGA AND BIO-PSYCHOLOGY	36
SHUKRA	37
THE MIND, YOGIC PRACTICE AND LYMPH	38
GLANDS	40
PINEAL GLAND	41
PITUITARY GLAND	42
THYROID AND PARATHYROID GLANDS	43
THYMUS GLAND	43
ADRENAL GLANDS	44
THE GONADS	44
YOGA PHYSIOLOGY	46
MUSCULAR SYSTEM	46
CIRCULATORY SYSTEM	47
SPINAL COLUMN	48
HEALTHY JOINTS	48
ÁSANAS, INTRODUCTION TO	50
1-LOTUS POSTURE - PADMÁSANA	52
2-BRAVE POSTURE - VIIRÁSANA	54
3-YOGAMUDRÁ - YOGAMUDRÁ	56
4-LONG BOWING POSTURE - DIIRGHA PRAŃÁMA	58
5-COBRA POSTURE - BHÚJAUNGÁSANA	60
6-BALANCE POSTURE - TULÁDANDÁSANA	63
7-LOCUST POSTURE - SHALABHÁSANA	64
8-BOAT POSTURE - NAOKÁSANA	66
9-WHEEL POSTURE - CAKRÁSANA	68

10-BELLOWS POSTURE	- BHASTRIKÁSANA	70
11-UTKŚEPA MUDRÁ	- UTKŚEPA MUDRÁ	71
12-HARE POSTURE	- SHASHÁUNGÁSANA	72
13-CAMEL POSTURE	- UŚTRÁSANA	74
14-THUNDER POSTURE	- VAJRÁSANA	76
15-THUNDER POSTURE, DIFFICULT	- UTKAŤA VAJRÁSANA	77
16-COW'S HEAD POSTURE	- GOMUKHÁSANA	78
17-BOUND LOTUS POSTURE	- BADDHA PADMÁSANA	80
18-HEAD TO KNEE POSTURE	- JÁNUSHIRÁSANA	82
19-FULLHEAD TO KNEE POSTURE	- PASHCIMOTTÁNÁSANA	84
20-FOOT TO HEAD POSTURE	- EKAPADASHIIRŚÁSANA	86
21- SPINAL TWIST	- MATSYENDRÁSANA	88
22- ALL LIMBS POSTURE	- SARVÁUNGÁSANA	90
23- FISH GESTURE	- MATSYAMUDRÁ	92
24- THE PLOUGH	- HALÁSANA	94
25- TREE POSTURE	- VRKŚÁSANA	96
26- JOINT LOOSENING POSTURE	- GRAŃTHIMUKTÁSANA	98
27- SHIVÁSANA	- SHIVÁSANA	100
28- SHAVÁSANA	- SHAVÁSANA	101

SOME COMMON GUIDELINES FOR
NATURAL AND HEALTHY LIVING ... 102
    EARTH ... 103
    WATER ... 103
    SUNBATH ... 104
    AIR, AIR-BATH ... 105
THE VEGETARIAN PYRAMID ... 106
FOOD ... 107
REFLEXOLOGY ... 108
SYSTEM FOR PRACTICING
YOGA ÁSANAS ... 110
ANTI-AGING: LONGEVITY PROGRAM ... 113
ÁSANAS TABLE ... 114
    ÁSANAS IN STANDING POSITION ... 114
    ÁSANAS IN SITTING POSITION ... 120
    ÁSANAS ON THE FLOOR ... 122
SAMSKRTA GLOSSARY ... 124

INDEX
For diseases with the number of the ásanas

abdominal muscles, strengthens **24**
abdominal problems **5, 1**
acidity **7, 15, 19**
acne, good for **23**
adrenal glands, balances **8**
anaemia **22**
appendicitis **19, 23**
appetite, increases **8, 16**
arm muscles, strengthens **8, 17**
arthritis **16, 26**
arthritis, pain in back **21**
asthma **8, 13, 23, 1**
attentive capacity, increases **26**
aura, creates **9**

back muscles, strengthens **27**
back, stretches **25**
back, supple **12, 15**
backbone, strengtens **20**
backpain **13, 15, 16**
bile production, balances **13**
blood circulation in legs, increases **7**
blood circulation in uterus
      for easier delivery, **5**
blood circulation, good for **4**
body and mind balance **25, 26**
body balance, maintains **20**
body, energises **20**
body, keeps flexible **20**
body, tones up **24**
bowels, cleanses **10, 11**
breathing, deeper **4, 5, 13, 23, 25**

cakras, activates **21**
calcification **9,**
calcification in vertebrae, prevents **21**
calcium, maintains in the body **23**
calmness, brings **21**
celibacy, helps maintain **13**
cellulite **7**
chest, made beautiful **8, 9**
chest, opens **17**
cholera, good for **22**
circulation of energy **13**
cold pox, relieves **22**
colic pain **18**
compression in nerves **19**
concentration, increases **25, 1**
constipation **4, 5, 7, 9, 10, 13,**
      16, 21, 22, 23, 24

depression, relieves **1**
diabetes **9, 13, 15, 19**
digestion **2, 15, 18, 19**
dyspepsia **16, 21, 8**

elbows, good for **26**
endocrine glands, stimulates **1**
excess fat reduces around the hips **7**
eye disorders **2**
eyesight, improves **13**

fatigue, removes **27**
fear **8**
fear, removes **2**
feminine disorders **1**
filthy thoughts, removes **16**

gas, removes **10, 23**
glands, activates **22**
glands, rests **22**
glow, creates **9**
gout **8, 14, 16**
gout in hands and feet **7**
gout in joints **26**
grey hair, stops growth of **13**
gums and teeth, proper
      blood circulation **23**

handmuscles, strengthens **16, 17**
hands and feet, made flexible **20**
harsh voice, softens **13**
headache **13, 22**
heart, good for **3, 5, 10, 16, 28**
hernia **22, 23**
high blood pressure, good for **28**
hormone secretion, increases **20**
hyperactive tendency, removes **20**

idleness, removes **17, 18**
impotency **1, 9**
indigestion **8, 9, 24**
insomnia **16, 1**
intestinal diseases **10, 11**
intestines, activates **8**
intuition, increases **2**

joints, works strongly **26**

kidneys, good for **16, 18, 20**
knees, flexible **19, 26**

laziness **8, 17**
leg muscles, strengtens **8, 20**
leprosy **8, 22**
lethargy **17**
leucoria **22**
liver, spleen, pancreas, good for **3, 4, 19, 21, 22, 24, 27**
longevity, creates **14, 22**
lower back pain **9, 13, 18, 21, 24**
lung capacity, increases **9, 13, 17**
lungs, strengtens **7, 8, 16**

meditation, beneficial for **3, 12, 1, 18**
memory power, increases **12, 24, 1**
menopause, good for **23**
menstruation pain, prevents **4, 5, 7, 22**
mental peace, brings **21**
mental work, good for **1**
metabolism, increases **20**
migraine
mind, active **17**
mind, relaxes **28**

neck troubles **13**
neckpain, in beginning of **24**
nerves and veins of stomach, strengtens **4, 5, 18**
nerves and veins, strengtens **12, 26**
nerves in back, massages **8**
nervous system, rejuvenates **26**

obesity **3, 4, 5, 9, 12, 17, 19, 24**

pancreas, balances hormones **12, 15, 23**
parathyroid gland, balances hormones **23**
patience, increases **24, 8**
patience, develops **8**
phlegm, removes **13**
piles **3, 16, 18, 19, 22**
pineal gland, effect on **24**
pneumonia **22**
psychic ailments, relieves **1**
psycho-physical pain **19**

rheumatism **7, 9, 16**
rheumatism, muscular **24**

scattered mind **6**
sciatica **14, 16, 18, 19**
self-confidence, increases **17**
sharpens the intellect **2**
shooting pain, relieves **22**
shoulder muscles, strengthens **16**
shoulder troubles **13**
skin diseases **23**
sleep, excessive **22**
spine, balanced **22**
spine, rejuvenates **21**
spine, stretches **9, 19, 24**
spine, strong and flexible **9, 13, 14, 16, 17**
spleen, good for **8**
stress **8**
stunted growth, helps to fight **9, 13**
syphilis **8**

tension **8**
thymus gland, balances hormones **18**
thyroid gland, balances hormones **12, 22**
tolerate cold and heat **13**
tonsilitis **12, 22**
toxins in back, removes **8**
toxins in cartildages, removes **4**
toxins of limbs, clears **26**
toxins stuck in body, removes **13**

upper legs, strengthens **7**
urinary duct, burning sensation **16**
uterus, displaced **22**

veins and nerves of back, strengthens **5**
vertebrae, exercises **13, 24**
vertebrae, massages **16**
vishuddha cakra **23**
vital fluids, flowing **1**
vitality of life, creates **4**
vitality, increases **26**
vocal cord, strengtens **23**

will power, increases **1, 3**
wind, releases trapped **7, 13**
wrist and arm muscles, strengthens **16**

youthfulness, keeps **14**

PREFACE

I am not a born yogi. By His cosmic plan, I came to the path of yoga in my teens. So eventually, yoga became my path and yoga became my goal. Since my adolescence, I have been practicing yoga, as a way or a style of life. Of course, it is a long way. While treading this path of eternal happiness, one passes through inummerable experiences, unbelievable happenings and extraordinary incidents.

To achieve the goal through this path is not to make castles in the sky. It is within our reach. If you have a real desire for it then you will achieve the goal, this is certain. However, you must have that irresistible desire to extend your hands and mind in order to find your true self.

My earnest request is, that nobody should shudder to think that yoga practice is a very difficult and dangerous affair. This whole book conveys this message; if you put forth a sincere effort, you can do Yoga in your own home by following the instructions contained here. Of course it is also recommended that you seek the guidance of a competent teacher, and use his or her instructions to compliment the teachings you find here.

The practice of Yoga is easy and the results are permanent. It is so simple that one needs nothing but a corner of a room, and the desire to do it. We have to remember that we, as human beings, do so many things for others and for society but often do little or nothing for ourselves. Yoga is your own thing. This practice, which is so beneficial and natural, must and should be done regularly. Once you practice Yoga the result is "in your pocket", this is my belief. Since this is the case, and these practices offer so many benefits to anyone who approaches them with sincerity, it is my humble request that everyone should have the opportunity to experience these benefits for themselves by following the path of Yoga outlined here.

I had never thought to write a book before. Many students who attended my classes in Istanbul, Turkey were constantly requesting that I write a book so that they might have a reference for the methods and aspects of Yoga I was teaching.

As I conducted my research into the Yoga books currently on the market; I noticed that very few addressed the scientific aspects of Yoga. Yoga has it's own special guidelines, which make these practices both rare and transcendent. Very few authors have acknowledged Yoga's vast spiritual dimensions.

Through the students constant determined demands and the invaluable assistance of Kalyáńii who helped to translate the essays I had hand-written over the years from English to Turkish, the first book was created. In this book I addressed the practice of Yoga, not only for the physical benefits or mental dynamism it creates, but also for the spiritual enlightenment it provides. This spiritual advancement will help all of humanity build an integrated personality and a dynamic society to meet the challenges of the twenty first century.

As a Yoga teacher, working for more than thirty-five years around the world, I have found the practice and philosophy of Yoga to be a binding force for the entire human race. This is because Yoga goes beyond any narrow outlook and is truly universal.

During the last four or five years, there has been a tremendous interest in Yoga all over the world, and as a result I have had to travel quite extensively.

Once I happened to carry my book to one of our yoga centers, in Sweden. The practitioners of that center who are very close to me, with whom I have passed many days and nights, wanted the book translated into English.

As we say, so we do. Yoga has a cosmic spirit. It brings about union and wonder.

A yogi never knows, where he or she will be tomorrow!

We began immediately. From experience we have learned, if we delay a project it will never be finished. Also procrastination is not consistent with a yogic way of life!

So it is not an exaggeration to say: We made the impossible, possible.

While continuing their daily routine, they were able to compose the book in English in seven days. It was through an extraordinary commitment, indomitable spirit, and untiring effort that we were able to compose the book you have before you in this short span of time.

These brothers and sisters are very near and dear to me and I don't know what to offer them to show them the depths of my appreciation for there untiring efforts. Of course I would not be satisfied to just convey my thanks. That word seems wholly inadequate to express my gratitude to my dear ones. Simply, I would like to mention their names as without their sincere, loving, enthusiastic help, I am sure I would never have completed this book in such a short period of time.

Saomyamúrti, from England, encouraged me to go ahead and later helped by translating and typing the benefits. Jitendriya, from Australia, who in the first instance approached me with the idea to publish the book in English, eventually went through the whole book and gave the proper shape to it. Sandiipan, from Argentina; together with Hanumanjii "Charles Brumley" from USA and Cirainjiiv from Turkey, who came voluntarily, developed the media and completely changed the sound, colour, form and vibration of the whole book. Our silent brother Pránesha from Brazil, who was an unseen force in the production! Sisters Sánanda from Sweden and Puńyáshiila from Vietnam, Hatice Öcal, Ümran Yeğin Uśa, Özlem Dokur and İnci Evrensel from Turkey gave the final touches. Also, I can't help admiring Arundhatii's (from Turkey) courage and efficiency for performing all the yogic postures in the book.

Last but not least I'd like to thank all the brothers and sisters, and the ashramites who came from all over the world and helped by giving their positive vibration and through their silent cooperation and smiling faces

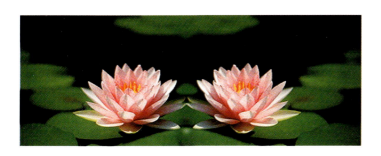

INTRODUCTION

In Yoga, practice precedes theory. The practice of Yoga goes beyond the utterance of theory alone. It is the systematic approach that allows us to achieve a successful result. The realised yogis achieved deep practical experience out of their spontaneous effort to find reality in themselves. The ancient yogis and munis (saints) observed the movement of flora and fauna – the animals and environment, and experimented with human nature. By this method, they discovered the science of Yoga. This deep mind and subtle realisation made a mark in the sciences of Physiology and Psychology.

Over hundreds of years or even millennia of practice the postures and gestures evolved. Gradually it became part of the behaviour in the body-mind of human beings, generation after generation. This is how thousands of yoga postures came into existence. All these movements are called the ásanas. Amongst the thousands of ásanas there are many which are good for both the physical body and mind, which are helpful for the psychology and morality of a person. If someone practices these ásanas for several hours, one will not get tired. Rather, one will feel more introverted, calm and quiet. So, all these selected ásanas are not only for the spine, vertebrae, bones or muscles, although the latter will certainly be benefited. Ásanas also help the inner organs to function properly. Most internal influences take place via the action of the endocrine glands, whose secretion of hormones has profound effects on the body-mind.

To be successful in yoga practices one should pay particular attention to certain key aspects: first,

Áhára – proper and healthy food; second,

Bihára – proper and healthy thoughts; and third,

Vyavahára – proper and healthy behaviour.

The material that makes up our cells is derived from the food we eat and drink. The thoughts that occupy our mind also form what we are. Hence, as you think so you become. The conclusion is that the neuro-chemical impulses of the nervous system and the biochemical signalling of our glandular system have an integral relationship with the way food, thought and behaviour are expressed in the body and mind. Through Yoga we can utilise an understanding of this relationship to create overall health, well-being and fulfilment of our human potential.

The science of Yoga tells us what to eat, how to eat, which foods to eat and in which ways the foods will affect our bodies and our minds. In our life, our behaviour will reflect the food we eat and our thoughts. Yoga influences the neuro-chemical signals and balance of the brain. Confusion, complexity, depression, extreme tension or extreme behaviour, absence of mental peace, anxiety, anger... all these can be changed by practicing yoga. These negative thoughts and emotions are the things that poison our life. By practicing Yoga one can achieve a balanced, calm, and focused mind, free from these negative thoughts and emotions.

The ásanas can impact the glands by causing them to secrete positive hormones. Ásanas also make the bones and muscles strong. They help to correct one's physical posture, to promote proper breathing and through their practice one can know how to store energy and maximize its use. One becomes physically relaxed and healthy – mentally tranquil and full of vigour.

As Rája Yoga gives stress or importance to Manah Shuddhi (purification of mind), Hatha Yoga (Yoga Ásanas) gives importance to Deha Shuddhi (the purification of the body). According to Hatha Yoga, one cannot accomplish Manah Shuddhi without Deha Shuddhi. Surely our body (deha) is the base of sádhaná (meditation practice). If we do not make our main base strong and stout we cannot build up the base of our life divine. Our body is like an instrument behind which there is the átma (spirit or soul). The átma is the permanent unseen guide and invisible force, which leads this sound body towards the door of sound and sublime mind, to allow it to reach the goal of attaining Cosmic Energy or Consciousness.

If the different aspects of the human body function properly and naturally, automatically the inherent divinity will be expressed through that body. On the contrary, if parts of the body are not functioning properly, the same human being can become the victim of ugly instincts, which turn a human being into an animal in human disguise. As for example, if the pituitary gland is not functioning correctly, one lacks magnanimity of mind, becomes narrow minded, wants to find fault or defects in others, tends to cruelty and engages in exploiting others. We may think that a person is bad, but in fact he or she is helpless. Several body mechanisms are under the influence of the hormone secretion, so, bad thoughts and negative activities are unwillingly being nourished and performed by the person. It is a similar case with other glands and cakras. Every cakra has both positive and negative vrttis (psycho-physical propensities, or tendencies).

By Hatha Yoga one can channelize and sublimate the baser vrtiis and tendencies towards higher pursuits. Cakras in the body are simply the conjoining points of different nerves, nerve cells and glands. If there is no proper glandular secretion from the fourth Cakra (Anáhata), there will be disturbance in the third Cakra (Manipura). As the Anáhata controls the aerial factor in the body, the Manipura controls the luminous factor. In the same way that a light extinguishes in a closed pot without air, so the life of the lamp becomes dim, if the air controller, the fourth cakra, does not function properly. I mean to say that there is a happy blending between the glands – and the harmony of the cells, the body-mind and nervous system depends on it.

The nervous system of the body is one of the most complex and wonderful phenomenon in the human structure. The entire machine of the body is operated by the nerves, or the central nervous system. The center of the central nervous system is the brain. Whatever order is given by the brain and transmitted through the nerves, the body carries it out by means of different nerve cells, which carry the order to the limbs. So the nerves or the nervous system directly or indirectly influences the nature of the body and mind of a human being. If the nerves and nerve fibres are not strong and lively, it affects the body and mind of a human being and as a result of that various psycho-physical problems arise. Only by performing yoga ásanas, meditation and the related rules and regulations, can one prevent oneself from developing any sort of unexpected or premature disease.

I will be very happy if people can apply these guidelines in their daily life to maintain good health, happiness and mental peace. In "Cure Yourself With Yoga" along with the yoga ásanas or postures, we will explain more on different features of the yogic lifestyle, summarized below:

1) Yoga exercises;
2) Proper nourishment (food);
3) Positive thinking;
4) Honest behaviour with oneself and the environment, while expressing both physically and mentally;
5) How to get into the flow of a natural lifestyle.

In this way by developing a proper psycho-chemical composition we can achieve a healthy mind-body. To achieve this goal is completely in our hands. With this positive mind and awakened spirit one easily treads the steps toward success. Whatever instincts we have that carry us towards negativity are hidden in human nature, and the same human being has the mind and rationality by which those undesirable tendencies can be transcended, releasing the person to move towards the fundamental positivity of life.

As a unified discipline, yoga aims at all-round development of an integrated personality. Step by step, it improves physical health, harmonizes thought and emotions and awakens the divine qualities.

I am sure that all who read and try to follow the guidance written in this book will derive maximum benefit from it.

It is my ardent desire to help people's well-being.

Let this book be a guiding light for genuine practitioners.

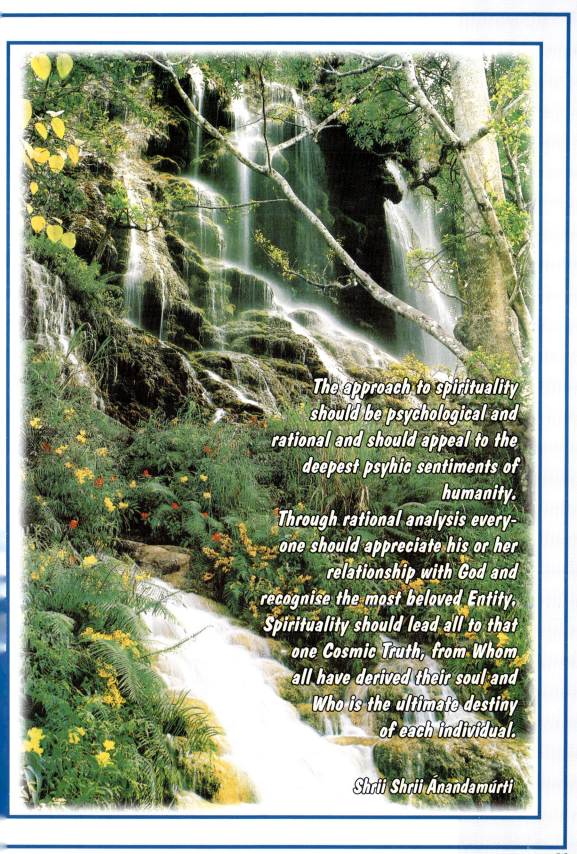

HISTORY

The historical origins of Yoga philosophy started thousands of years ago. Veda, the earliest scripture provides the knowledge of Yoga, which was traditionally transmitted orally through the ages; as it was not written in the days of yore. Later, with the passage of time, the Yoga we know today was developed as a part of the Tantrik Civilization, which existed in India and all parts of the world more than ten thousand years ago. In Tantra there is the concept of Shiva and Shakti. Shiva or Ádináth who is the primal master or protector, is the first leader of the human society who combined the methods of intuitional science, which later became known as Yoga, about 7000 years ago.

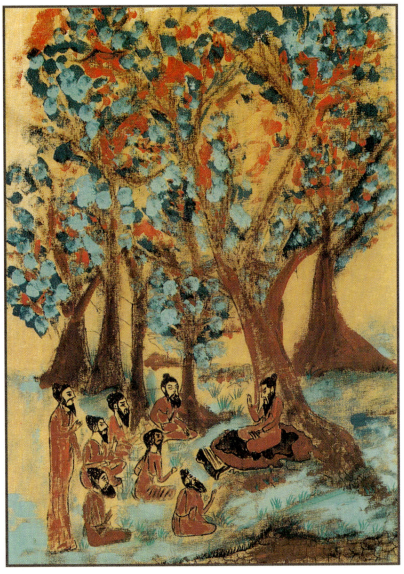

The practical spiritual cult, Tantra, is a combination of two words: TAN and TRA, which means 'expand' and 'liberate' respectively. It is the science of expanding one's consciousness, which is quiescent in every human being and liberates the energy in the physical, mental and spiritual spheres. Tantra is the way by which one can liberate oneself from these trifarious bondages and attain freedom from the bondage of the world while still living in it.

Around the 3rd Century BC a great sage named Pátainjali who was born at Pátun in Burdwan district, Bengal; composed his celebrated yoga sútras or aphorisms of yoga. Sage Pátainjali's treatise on Rája-Yoga, the yoga sútras, codifies the first definitive, unified and comprehensive system of Yoga.

Though the knowledge of Yoga had already existed for thousands of years before him, he is considered to be the first author who truly put the different aspects in order and systematized it theoretically.

The never-ending search for truth continued. The spiritual aspirants realized the effects of yoga on different glands and sub-glands, which are located in the main nerve centers at the point of each cakra. The sub-glands influence the propensities attached to each cakra. This is a new science which is still unknown today.

"The process of controlling all the cakras and the propensities was invented by Aśtávakra over 2000 years ago. He wrote the book Aśtávakra Samghitá. He was a great saint and called the process 'Rájádhirája Yoga'. He first taught this system of Yoga to Alarka at Vakreshwar in Bengal".

Shrii Shrii Ánandamúrti from "Yoga Psychology".

In the last century, Shrii Shrii Ánandamúrti, the Great Advent of the 20th century systematized, introduced and demonstrated the practical method of Rájádhirája Yoga for the entire human society. He trained hundreds of His disciples who are propagating His ideology throughout the world in order to help the suffering humanity by teaching all the aspects of Yoga.

Such is the origin and history of the ancient science of Yoga, which is a practical and profound spiritual discipline for all time throughout the world. Today in the 21st century, yoga is essential to obtain the highest goal of the spiritual path. However yoga is beneficial to everyone regardless of their spiritual aims.

In an age of technological achievements with computers, mobile phones and super-markets, yogic practices make great personal and business sense on the physical level. For having a dynamic and peaceful mind, the method of Aśtáunga Yoga is introduced, and for creating the final harmony between mind, body and spirit, the practice of Rájádhirája is the final goal.

The different aspects of yoga will be explained step by step:

Rájádhirája Yoga

Rájádhirája Yoga has eight steps to perfection. Yoga meditation is performed by the mind and a sound mind requires a sound body. For this reason, the Yoga ásanas play a very important role in the practice. In Aśtáunga Yoga, Yama-Niyama, which is a complete purification method for our mental and physical existence, is followed by ásana. Ásanas are innumerable in numbers. It would not be possible to find all of the ásanas that have been developed in one book, nor would there be time in one life to practice all of them.

Hence, those ásanas which are good for both mind and body, which can be performed easily or which are the most beneficial for curing many common diseases, have been serially elaborated in this book.

I would like to emphasize that, though several diseases can be cured by the practice of ásanas, cure is not the goal of ásanas. We should always bear in mind that prevention is better than cure. So, while practising, please take the ideation of your Supreme goal purely and with sincerity. In this way you wil develop a sound mind and a sound body for achieving the spiritual goal through yoga meditation.

Hatha Yoga-This yoga with physical gestures and postures is popularly known in the West. Hatha yoga is the first and foremost yoga known to the Western world. Usually a person comes to yoga to practice physical exercises that will help to bring proper hormone secretion and achieve a disease-free body. Kundalinii Yoga is another name, meaning to arouse the kula kundalinii energy within a human being. This energy is described as a "coiled serpentine force" lying dormant in the Múládhára cakra, in every human being. Yogic methods will help to arouse it, freeing its movement up through the spinal column.

Dhyána Yoga: The Samskrta word for meditation is dhyána. So Dhyána Yoga helps to learn different techniques of meditation. Often in Hatha Yoga classes people ask for instruction in the practice of meditation.

Rája Yoga – Yoga of inner concentration; where mind is concentrated towards the subjectivity of self.

Jinána Yoga – The yoga of intellect; yoga in the psychic sphere. It will help one to liberate, bringing one from the normal boundaries of the mind.

Bhakti Yoga – The yoga of perfect love, i.e. love for G.O.D. (the Generator, Operator and Destroyer), or Supreme Consciousness centred through an image or idea of divinity towards the created universe where the Divine is perceived through the idea of cosmic love. Bhakti yoga helps the sádhaka to unify with the Supreme.

Karma Yoga – Karma means action. When karma is done without being involved with transanctional mentality, one feels no attachment to the result of Karma. Whatever is done, it is done for the Divinity. While performing an action one surrenders and therefore doesn't receive the reaction of the performed action. While acting one should maintain in the mind the idea that we have the right to act only, and not the right to receive the result of the action. Humans are the machines and the unseen Supreme Entity is the machine-operator.

Similarly, there are so many other varieties of yoga, viz, Kriyá Yoga, Laya Yoga, Tapah Yoga, Siddhánta Yoga, Bháva Yoga, Abháva Yoga, Astáunga Yoga*, Náda Yoga, Bindu Yoga, Mahá Yoga, Sahaja Yoga, Ánanda Yoga, etc.

Rájádhirája Yoga combines all the important aspects of yoga, and guides the spiritual aspirant through each step in the process one after another. Its system will help one to accomplish the duties of the world and at the same time perform all the psycho-spiritual practices, keeping the hands to work and heart to Life Divine. It will make one physically fit, mentally strong, morally elevated and spiritually enlightened.

* For Astáunga yoga see page 30

ORIGINAL ALL-ROUND LIFE STYLE

THE TEACHINGS OF SHIVA

The practical spiritual cult, **Tantra**, the first methods of Intuitional Science, were taught by Shiva about 7000 years ago, later known as YOGA.

Around 2300 years ago Pátaińjali systematised **YOGA** with sútras. He was born at Pátun, Burdwan, Bengal. (INDIA)

Over 2000 years ago Aśtávakra Muni from Vakreshwar, Bengal taught **Rájádhirája yoga**, the practical yogic methods to his follower Alarka.

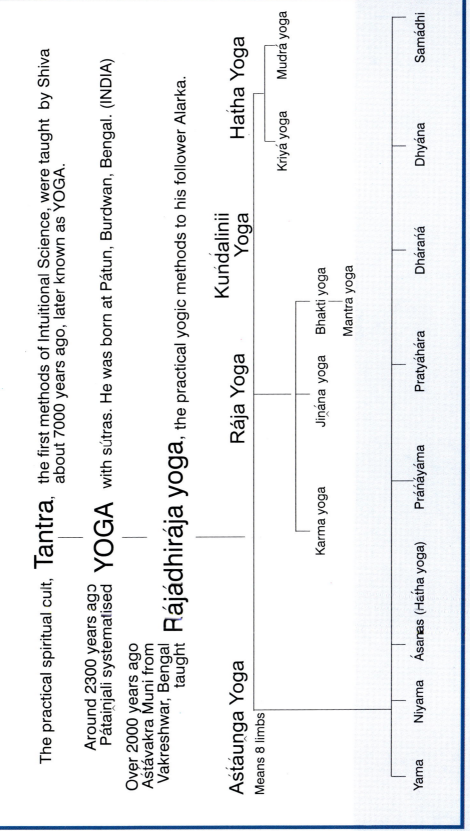

Aśtáunga Yoga
Means 8 limbs

- Rája Yoga
  - Karma yoga
  - Jińána yoga
  - Bhakti yoga
  - Mantra yoga
- Kuńdalinii Yoga
- Hatha Yoga
  - Kriyá yoga
  - Mudrá yoga

Yama — Niyama — Ásanas (Hatha yoga) — Práńáyáma — Pratyáhára — Dháraná — Dhyána — Samádhi

YOGA PHILOSOPHY

In the cycle of creation everything travels from subtle to crude and from crude to subtle. The wheel of creation emerges with varying shapes, varying bodies, varying forms and varying names. The different forms are called "rúpa", and the different names "náma".

We are in the labyrinth of this creative wheel taking different rúpas and námas.

Nothing is completely conscious or unconscious. Whether it is big or small, sentient or static, matter or spirit, conscious or superconscious, all is moving according to the plan of the cosmic consciousness.

Thus it is said that, this creation is nothing but the expression of the cosmic entity. That cosmic consciousness is called the bháva (idea) and this idea wants to take it's own expression, it's own rúpa. As the rúpa gradually crudifies and the rúpa can no longer remain bound, it searches for freedom.

But freedom from where? Are we born free? No; we come with fetters. They are our own bondages with our energy. The moment life comes with mind in this creation, it gets three constituents; ie. I exist, I do, and I am. Philosophically they are known as Mahattattva, Ahamtattva, and Cittatattva.

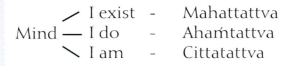

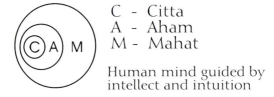

Human mind guided by intellect and intuition

While speaking about Mahattattva, Ahamtattva and Cittatattva, I have to mention more about the first basic proposition in Shrii Shrii Ánandamúrti's spiritual philosophy where Brahma or God is the composite of Puruśa and Prakrti; or the Cosmic Cognitive Principle, Cosmic Consciousness and the Cosmic Operative Principle or Cosmic Energy respectively.

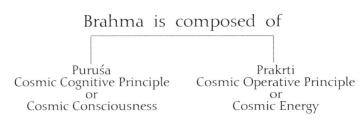

As with two sides of a piece of paper, these two cannot be separated from each other under any circumstances. Puruśa is the Cosmic Witness, the all-pervasive consciousness quiescent in each and every entity. Prakrti is the attribute of Puruśa and is a belligerent force. When Puruśa manifests itself Prakrti is dominant, out of His desire. Prakrti binds Puruśa resulting in the manifestation of the Cosmic Mind and the universe. The stage of Brahma where Puruśa is desireless and has no will and Prakrti is unexpressed is called Nirguńa Brahma. The stage of Brahma where Puruśa comes under the bondages of Prakrti, because Puruśa desires it, is known as Saguńa Brahma.

We the human beings, as practitioners of meditation make all-round effort to be in Nirguńa Brahma with one-pointed and concentrated thinking and as a result of that one attains the balance of mind where one goes beyond the torments of pleasure and pain. One liberates oneself from the world of bondages. Liberation is the final and ultimate goal of life.

Everyone longs and strives for true happiness, wants to break the walls of limitations of conditioned existence. Real happiness, Ánandam the eternal Bliss and unending peace can be obtained only when the soul is freed from all bondages.

Very few people seek happiness by way of following the natural and sentient rules for mind and body. Only by way of disciplining the body, mind and intellect, one can follow the path of Rájádhirája Yoga. Rájádhirája yoga alone will help one to break the bondages of limited Náma and Rúpa and merge oneself in the highest level of pure consciousness (Bháva). The long journey will end with the final destination.

Brahma Cakra

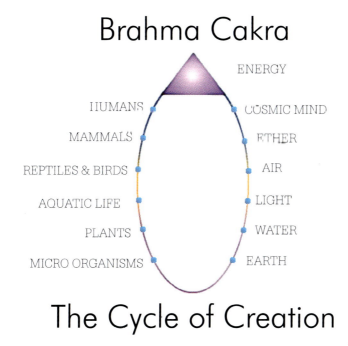

The Cycle of Creation

CAKRAS AND KOŚAS

The science of Yoga is for everyone in this world, irrespective of caste, creed, colour, nationality, sex etc. Yoga is a practice for the entire humanity. One has the birthright to practice yoga. The first awareness we have is that we are human. Human beings possess both instinct and rationality. It is the rational mind which discriminates between right and wrong. One of the main characteristics of humans is that we can think carefully with concentration. This can lead one to meditation. Meditation is a concentrated thought method. This thinking process is bound to various cakras or plexi – the name for specific collections of glands and subglands. Cakras are the psychic centres of the body through which energy flows. In addition to the cakras, there are three major energy channels called Iidá, Piuṇgalá and Suśumńá nádiis. Nádiis are the energy channels, and where these three energy channels intersect with each other lie the cakras. Our body's nervous system is also intimately connected with to the network of nádiis.

The human body is a biological machine. Those who want to tread the path of spirituality must use this machine with proper thinking, feeling, and decision making, by utilizing the thoughts, which constantly emerge and dissolve, in a proper way. Underlying these psychic phenomena are our reactive momenta, or saḿskáras. The saḿskáras can be described as the accumulated reactions of our past actions (karma) in potential form. The vrttis (mental propensities) are formed according to one's saḿskáras.

The vrttis of the human being express and control the secretions of hormones from different glands and sub-glands located near the different cakras.

The following chart shows the names of different cakras in the human structure, the elements they control and the mańdalas or circles, which surround them:

Name of the elements	Name of the cakras	Name of the mańdalas
Terranean plexus	Múládhára	Bhaoma Mańdala
Fluidal plexus	Svádhiśthána	Tarala Mańdala
Igneous plexus	Mańipura	Agni Mańdala
Solar plexus	Anáhata	Saora Mańdala
Sidereal plexus	Vishuddha	Nakśatra Mańdala
Lunar plexus	Ájiná	Candra Mańdala

Corresponding to the first five cakras, there are five layers of mind, known as kośas. According to yoga, expansion is life and contraction is death – so if we want to live like a divine human being we have to go through an expansion process from lower or crude levels of mind to subtler levels. As one's mind becomes more elevated, it passes through higher, more subtle layers of consciousness or kośas.

According to one's level of mental elevation, a consciousness of the five layers of existence may arise. This consciousness is known as paiṅca kośa viveka

With the help of paiṅca kośa viveka ('the conscience of five layers of existence') people can easily discern that the :

Annamaya Kośa — (physical body);
Kámamaya Kośa — (crude mind);
Manomaya Kośa — (subtle mind);
Atimánasa Kośa,
Vijiṅánamaya Kośa, — (causal mind)
Hirańmaya Kośa

are separate layers; that consciousness is above all five kośas. Spiritual Sádhaná (spiritual meditation) means ideation on one's own consciousness beyond these kośas and not ideation on any of these kośas themselves.

Cakras
Centers of Energy

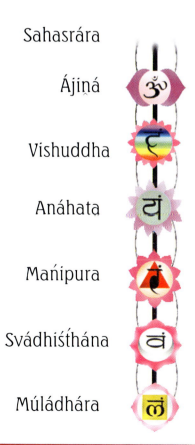

Sahasrára

Ájiṅá

Vishuddha

Anáhata

Mańipura

Svádhiśthána

Múládhára

THE RELATIONSHIP BETWEEN KOŚAS AND CAKRAS

Cakras play an important role in our psychic and psycho-spiritual development. While making the journey towards the Supreme Consiousness, one has to refine the body and mind through the cakras and their associated layers (kośas).

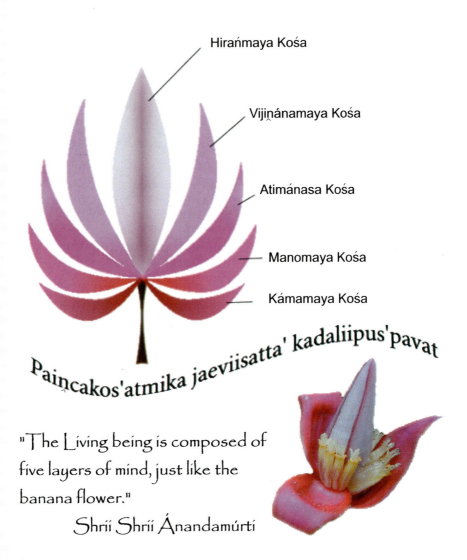

- Hirańmaya Kośa
- Vijiṅánamaya Kośa
- Atimánasa Kośa
- Manomaya Kośa
- Kámamaya Kośa

Paiṅcakos'atmika jaeviisatta' kadaliipus'pavat

"The Living being is composed of five layers of mind, just like the banana flower."

        Shrii Shrii Ánandamúrti

Following is the table for comparing their relationship;

Name of the kośas	Cakra relation	Layers of mind
Kámamaya kośa	Múládhára	Conscious mind
Manomaya kośa	Svádhiśthána	Sub-conscious mind
Atimánasa kośa	Mańipura	Supra-mental mind
Vijińánamaya kośa	Anáhata	Subliminal mind
Hirańmaya kośa	Vishuddha	Subtle causal mind

- *Annamaya Kośa*

The Samskrta word anna means food. The body is formed through food. So, Annamaya Kośa is the physical body.

- *Kámamaya Kośa*

The mind works behind the body. The mind is formed by Kámamaya Kośa. Káma means to desire. It is known as the crude mental body. The desires of the mind activate the sensory organs by stimulating them, and act to materialise the expected desires through motor organs and vrttis.

"Above the Kámamaya kośa there is an ordinary mind, which is created by the Manomaya Kośa. Confinement to the Annamaya Kośa tends to crudify a person since it doesn't allow for psychic elevation. Where the Annamaya Kośa dominates, all the remaining kośas are dormant."

- *Manomaya Kośa*

One experiences pain and pleasure and contemplates in this kośa. The memory and phenomena of dreams also occur in this layer.

- *Atimánasa Kośa*

One accumulates the samskáras in this kośa. One can develop intuition and creativity here. Telepathy, precognition, extra-sensory perception, clairvoyance etc. are the outcome of this kośa.

- *Vijińánamaya Kośa*

One gets Viveka and Vaerágya – Viveka means spiritual discrimination and Vaerágya means non-attachment. The storage of the seeds of samskáras lies here.

- *Hirańmaya Kośa*

This is the gateway to enter into the realm or kingdom of pure and Supreme Consciousness. So, the feeling of pure expression of "I exist" begins from this kośa.

The journey on the path of eternal bliss is a gradual and steady process based on Tantra. Tantra is a constant, systematic and regular practice that brings the sádhaka (spiritual practitioner) towards the ultimate goal of self-realization, by purification and transformation of the mind from the first kośa to the higher kośas. So, there is a corresponding link between the Aśtáunga yoga practice and the development of the kośas. By incorporating the unique practice of Yoga, based on Tantra, into our personal life we are attempting to reach the sublime state of spiritual awareness, which is the divine goal of each person who practices meditation. This is a state of peace, joy and complete well-being.

Throughout the spinal chord from top to bottom these five cakras are related to the 5 layers of mind, which also control five elements in the body, i.e earth, water, fire, air and ether. Up above the 5th cakra, which is related to Hirańmaya Kośa, there is the 6th cakra, named Ájiṋá Cakra. This cakra is beyond the reach of crude aspects of mind, i.e the five fundamental factors. It is the seat of the mind between the eyebrows, also called Trikuti.

Blind belief is not the goal of a true spiritual aspirant, instead one seeks to experience for themselves the truth of the teachings of Yoga. As the spiritual aspirant progresses in his or her practice they move beyond the realm of the individual mind to the 7th cakra, known as Sahasrára Cakra which is located 10 fingers above Ájiṋá Cakra. This is the place where one experiences the feeling of infinite bliss. One tastes the sweetness of divine nectar through all the levels of created consciousness. Out of that intoxication of divine nectar one starts dancing, smiling, crying and jumping. One gets beyond oneself with infinite joy, dipped in the ocean of Supreme Consciousness. The people in the world name them "the mad ones". This eternal feeling of boundless happiness, this supreme touch of that invisible force, this divine elixir from an unseen guide, this constant love, touch, sound and vision brings one beyond the periphery of religious dogma and belief.

One goes beyond the boundary of name, fame, dress, address and sits beside the ocean of the entire humanity singing the eternal song of spiritual enlightenment with the music of cosmic love. While being established in this highest Cakra, one is united with Cosmic bliss. That is the ultimate goal, the aim of human beings on this barren earth!

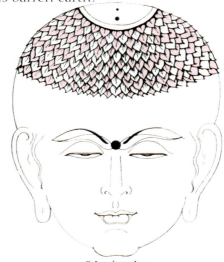

Sahasrára cakra

AŚTÁUNGA YOGA AND KOŚA

In short, yoga means, Aśtáunga yoga, but this concept tends to be misunderstood and followed in an incomplete manner. The path of yoga is often followed solely as Hatha yoga and Aśtáunga yoga which is thaught of as merely the name of some sort of yoga technique. If we really want to follow yoga in a true sense, we have to go through all the different aspects of Aśtáunga yoga.

'Aśta' means eight and 'aunga' means limbs of the body, we can say the eight hands of yoga. Therefore, if one wants to reach the goal of yoga, one has to follow, the 8 different aspects of yoga completely and fully. It is a step-by-step method. One cannot start doing everything simultaneously. In order to perform the steps of Aśtáunga yoga perfectly one needs the guidance of competent teachers. You will definitely find a teacher in your area, provided you have an irresistible desire to begin this practise. The disciples of Gurudeva Shrii Shrii Ánandamúrtijii are always available everywhere in the world, to help you wholeheartedly.

In the first step of Aśtáunga yoga one has to be a moralist. Without morality the foundation of spiritual growth will be very weak. And where there is weakness, there is stagnancy, no progress. The moral principels of Yama and Niyama are the foundation of one's spiritual journey and practice.

> By performing Ásanas, one purifies the body.
> Pránáyáma is the technique for controlling vital energy.
> Pratyáhára is the method to withdraw the mind and merge in His beauty.
> Dháraná is the ideation at a fixed point.
> Dhyána is the constant concentration with supreme ideation. It gives access to the soul.
> Samádhi – One looses one's barrier of pain and pleasure. One remains beyond the existence of unit consciousness.

By means of this Aśtáunga yoga, one can make the Paiṋca kośa (five layers of the mind) perfected. Pious persons are those who are sincere in their efforts to perfect the paiṋca kośa. So, human existence consists of the five kośas and spiritual practice is eightfold. This spiritual practice is the Dharma (characteristic) of human beings.

Names of the kośas	Aśtáunga Yoga techniques
Annamaya kośa	Ásana
Kámamaya kośa	Yama – Niyama
Manamaya kośa	Pránáyáma
Atimánasa kośa	Pratyáhára
Vijiṋánamaya kośa	Dháraná
Hiraṅmaya kośa	Dhyána

MÚLÁDHÁRA CAKRA

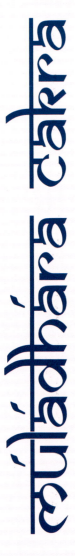

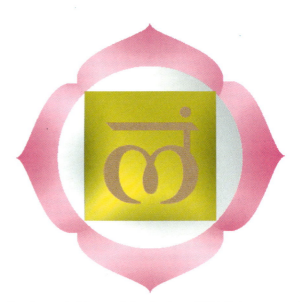

This is the fundamental base of the body – Múládhára means fundamental base. This is the place where the kuńdalinii lies dormant. The whole of human potentiality lies latent in this cakra.

Meaning of the word	: "Fundamental base"
Also known as	: Terranean plexus, root cakra
Position	: Coccyx bone of the spine
Form	: Square
Colour	: Golden yellow
Elements	: Earth, solid factor
Vibrational media (tanmátra)	: Smell
Properties related to other cakras	: Svádhiśthána – taste
	Mańipura – sight, vision
	Anáhata – touch
	Vishuddha – hearing, auditory

The four petals represent four different vrttis (propensities) of the mind that are controlled by this cakra.

Vrttis being controlled:

1- **Dharma** : psycho-spiritual longing
2- **Artha** : psychic longing
3- **Káma** : physical longing
4- **Mokśa** : spiritual longing

SVÁDHIŚŤHÁNA CAKRA

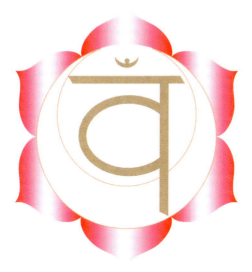

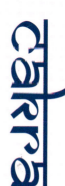

This cakra makes one strong, providing control over oneself. During human life many challenges arise. The strengthening of this cakra can help one to overcome these obstacles.

Meaning of the word	: Seat of my own energy.
Also known as	: Fluidal plexus
Position	: At the root of the sex organ
Form	: Crescent moon
Colour	: White
Elements	: Liquid
Vibrational media (tanmátra)	: Taste
Properties related to other cakras	: Manipura – sight, vision
	Anáhata – touch
	Vishuddha – hearing, auditory

The six petals represent the six vrttis of the Svádhiśťhána.

Vrttis being controlled:
1- **Avajiṅá** : belittlement of others
2- **Múrcchá** : psychic stupor, lack of common sense
3- **Prashraya** : indulgence
4- **Avishvása** : lack of confidence
5- **Sarvanásha**: thought of sure annihilation
6- **Krurata** : cruelty

MAŃIPURA CAKRA

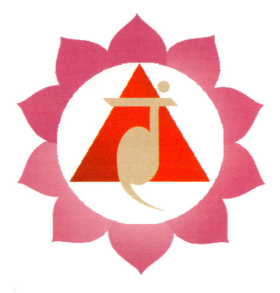

While passing through this cakra one develops great intellectual capacity. Intellectuality merges with intuition.

Meaning of the word	: This is the treasure house of the devotee.
Also known as	: Igneous plexus
Position	: Navel
Form	: Triangular
Colour	: Red
Elements	: Fire
Vibrational media (tanmátra)	: Heat
Properties related to other cakras	: Anáhata – touch
	Vishuddha – hearing, auditory

The ten petals of the lotus represent the expression of ten different vrttis.

Vrttis being controlled:

1- **Lajjá**	:	shyness, shame
2- **Piśhunatá**	:	sadistic tendency
3- **Íirśá**	:	envy
4- **Suśupti**	:	staticity, sleepiness
5- **Viśáda**	:	melancholia
6- **Kaśáya**	:	peevishness
7- **Trśńá**	:	yearning for acquisition
8- **Moha**	:	infatuation
9- **Ghrńá**	:	hatred, revulsion
10- **Bhaya**	:	fear

ANÁHATA CAKRA

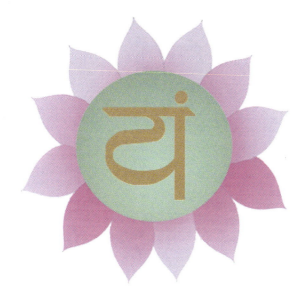

One receives preparation from this Cakra to listen to the Cosmic AUM with the inner ear.

Meaning of the word	: "Unstruck holy sound"
Also known as	: Solar plexus
Position	: Center of chest, heart
Form	: Circle
Colour	: Smoky colour
Elements	: Air
Vibrational media (tanmátra)	: Touch
Properties related to other cakras	: Vishuddha – hearing, auditory

The twelve petals of this lotus represent the twelve vrttis of the Anáhata.

Vrttis being controlled:

1- **Áshá**	:	hope
2- **Cíntá**	:	worry
3- **Ceśtá**	:	effort
4- **Mamatá**	:	mine-ness, love
5- **Dambha**	:	vanity
6- **Viveka**	:	conscience, discrimination
7- **Vikalatá**	:	mental numbness due to fear
8- **Ahamkára**	:	ego
9- **Lolatá**	:	avarice
10- **Kapatatá**	:	hypocrisy
11- **Vitarka**	:	argumentativeness to point of wild exaggeration
12- **Anutápa**	:	repentance

VÍSHUDDHA CAKRA

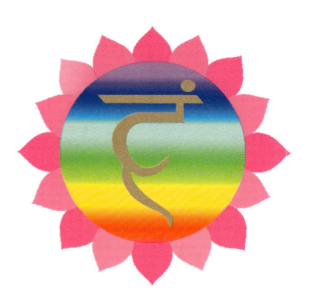

This cakra makes one free from wordly desires by bringing the sádhaka closer to the path of complete knowledge, which can only be achieved by increased concentration.

Meaning of the word	: Spotless purity
Also known as	: Sidereal plexus
Position	: Throat
Form	: Formless
Colour	: All colours
Elements	: Ether
Vibrational media (tanmátra)	: Hearing, auditory

The sixteen petals of this lotus represent the sixteen vrttis of the Vishuddha cakra.

Vrttis being controlled:

1- Śadaja	: sound of peacock
2- Rśabha	: sound of bull or ox
3- Gándhára	: sound of goat
4- Madhyama	: sound of deer
5- Paiṅcama	: sound of cuckoo
6- Dhaevata	: sound of donkey
7- Niśáda	: sound of elephant
8- Oṅm	: acoustic root of creation, preservation, dissolution
9- Hummm	: sound of arousing kulakun'd'alinii
10- Phat	: practication, i.e., putting a theory into practice
11- Vaośaṭ	: expression of mundane knowledge
12- Vaśaṭ	: welfare in the subtler sphere
13- Sváhá	: performing noble actions
14- Namah	: surrender to the Supreme
15- Viśa	: repulsive expression
16- Amrta	: sweet expression

ÁJÍŃÁ CAKRA

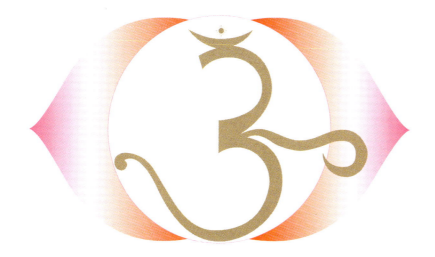

It is the place from where a person receives the knowledge of past, present and future. Such a person is called TRIKÁLAJIŃA. Who can see the three worlds, the past the present and the future.

Meaning of the word	: Authority, command, unlimited power
Location	: Point between the eyebrows
Also known as	: The third eye
Form	: Beyond form

It is subtler than the subtlest of the five elements and beyond the influence of the five fundamental factors. It is thus given as a point of concentration and iidá, puingalá and suśumńá conjoin. These three "rivers" meet in Triveńii, the main seat of consciousness. The third eye is the conscience. The two physical eyes see the past and the present, while the third eye reveals the insight of the future.

When one penetrates the sixth cakra one goes beyond the periphery of time, place and person. The duality between shiva and shakti, ying and yang and male and female energies ceases to exist. One remains only with one's Self.

The two lotus petals represent two propensities. The sádhaka has to discriminate and choose between Pará and Apará.
She or he, takes the decision to act either negatively or positively through this point.

Vrttís being controlled:

1- **Apará** : mundane knowledge
2- **Pará** : spiritual knowledge

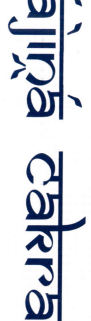

THE EIGHT STEPS OF SELF-REALISATION AŚTÁUNGA YOGA

According to yoga philosophy, this physical body is the machine and behind this ectoplasmic body, the soul or spirit is lying latent. So, the consciousness is ultimately the machine man. People often ask me whether I teach yoga or meditation. One should know that without a sound body, one cannot do proper meditation. The human body is only the base of meditation. When the nerves, veins, glands, muscles are normal in a body, then only can the divine in a human being arise in a proper way. If there is any defect in body-mind, the same human body becomes a base for suffering. For example, if someone does not work, he or she is likely to suffer from constipation and similar diseases, becomes peevish in nature, rough and cacophonic. If the thymus gland is inactive, one becomes cruel. If the pituitary gland does not work, one becomes narrow-minded, fault-finding, and jealous. So, if there is no purification of body, there is also no purification of the mind and heart!

Our human life can be considered with two major aspects. We have the innate quality of service – the human body wants to work to help it's own-self and others. It is the nature of the body to serve others.

Then comes the arena of mind. Mind can think, imagine and it has the tendency to be curious and to know the unknown. It wants to experience, to expand and satisfy the psychic pabula.

With a good body and good mind one possesses a good heart. One feels inspired to open their heart and embrace and love others. It is the nature of the heart to love others.

Conflict always remains between the body and mind, mind and heart, feeling and body. This conflict can only be overcome through the spirit of Devotion. Devotion is the attribute of soul. It is the nature of the soul to be one with the Cosmic Soul, the Supreme Soul. In every human being, there is a thirst – to be one with limitlessness.

No one becomes truly happy by satisfying physical desire, by experiencing pleasure only in the physical realm. According to human psychology, one wants more and more. This tendency can be fulfilled only with the infinite entity, so it is said: 'infinite pleasure is happiness'. That is the path of Ánanda, (Eternal Bliss). Each and every entity is moving towards that Ánanda. That path of eternal bliss is the path of Ánanda Márga; that is the Bhágavat Dharma. It is the path of eternity, the path of every human soul. Everybody, knowingly or unknowingly is searching for fulfilment on this level, everyone has an aspiration for this. YOGA encompassing Bhágavat Dharma, will help one to expand mentally, making one physically healthy, mentally balanced, morally strong and spiritually enlightened.

1. YAMA

Yama is comprised of the five principles by which we can maintain a harmonious existence with the external world. Living in accordance with these principles allows the mind to rise above the fetters of the mundane world. Yama therefore provides the basis for purity and clarity of mind through regulation of conduct, allowing us to attain higher levels of consciousness.

Yamas and Niyamas; restraints and observances forbid any kind of misuse of the potentiality of body and mind. Through their practice, one makes one's base strong for spirituality. These are the practical steps we can take to make our lives richer and more spirit-centered.

Yamas, the abstentions are:

"Ahim'sá": The word "Ahim'sá" means literally 'non-harm' (a:no , him'sá: harm). So, it means refraining from inflicting harm upon others without any reason.

"Satya": Satya is speaking the truth with the spirit of welfare

"Asteya": Asteya means non-stealing both physically and mentally. Withholding what is due to others also comes under Asteya.

"Brahmacarya": The word Brahma means Supreme Consciousness, so Brahmacarya means 'to follow God' who permeates every atom of the Universe.

"Aparigraha": It means a simple living without covetousness. While Brahmacarya is concerned with the subjective experience, Aparigraha is about our objective reality.

2. NIYAMA

The five principles of Niyama form part of the clear mental base that allows the aspirant to move towards subtler and deeper realisation. Niyama is concerned with our existence in the physical, mental and spiritual realms. The universal principles of Niyama offer a guidance for us in how to behave and guide our thinking to achieve mental peace. Niyama creates an integration of the personality. The things we think, we will speak and what we speak we will do – we will be consistent in thought and expression, reflecting inner and external balance.

Niyamas, the observances are:

"Shaoca": Shaoca or cleanliness is the first component of Niyama that is both external and internal, physical cleanliness and psychic cleanliness.

"Santośa": It means self-contentment that comes from accepting ourselves and others in the feeling of happiness. Without Santośa even a multimillionaire remains more unhappy than a begger.

"Tapah" : Tapah means austerity or penance. A conscious sacrificing practice of giving ourselves without any selfish motivation for reaching the goal.

" Service to humanity is service to God"

"Svádhyáya": To read those literatures that inspire and enlighten us. While reading the literatures and scriptures, one must use rational judgment in concert with feelings and intuition.

"Iishvara Prańidhána": The literal meaning of Iishvara Prańidhána is 'to take shelter in the Supreme'; which will help one to surrender the ego and live joyfully in the ups and downs of worldly life.

3. ÁSANAS
These are the yoga postures, which are explained in details on the blue pages ie. from page no.50.

4. PRÁŃÁYÁMA
It is the science of breathing. Práńa means vital energy; Ayáma means to regulate. The technique, by which we can get the maximum benefits out of our breath is the 'Práńáyáma system. Though there is not a single human being who can live without taking breath, still very few people know how to live with proper breathing. A human life is nothing but the parallelism of mind, body and práńendriya. If práńa leaves, the structure becomes a dead body. Similarly, the practice of proper breathing through práńáyáma makes one mentally healthy, concentrated and powerful. There are several práńáyáma techniques. One does not need to follow all of them. Práńáyáma should be learned not by books but through competent teachers. The science of práńáyáma is also called "Svarodaya Yoga"; the yoga system by which one knows the system of inhalation and exhalation. In our body there are different psychic energy channels, which are called nádiis. These nádiis are divided into three channels, Iidá, Piungalá and Suśumńá. If someone knows the technique to have control over and dominance over IIDÁ and Piungalá, and can understand the movement of inhalation and exhalation properly, one can live with a healthy and diseaseless body. Inhalation is called Púraka and exhalation is called Recaka. Holding the breathe in between is called Kumbhaka. Práńáyáma is very helpful for the practice of meditation (Dhyána) but one should not start it before completing the aforesaid parts of the 8-fold yoga-path (Aśt́áuŋga Yoga).

5. PRATYÁHÁRA
The word literally means 'withdrawal' - drawing back the unsteady and restless mind whenever it gets dispersed or loses focus. The best method and simplest means for withdrawal is to surrender everything at the feet of Guru through Varnághyadána, which is to be taught by the Ácáryas of Ánanda Márga yoga. We live in this phenomenal world, always occupied with the stimuli received by our senses. These are to be controlled and directed or sublimated towards Cosmic Consciousness by practising deep concentration and absorbing the mind in Him. Constant practice of Pratyáhára, by surrendering everything to the Cosmic Consciousness brings about the internalisation of the whole being – the attachment towards worldly things gradually transforms towards the attraction of the Great.

In Pátaiṇjali Darshan it is said,

"Sva-Visayasamprayoge cittasya svarúpánukara ekendriyáńáḿ pratyáhára".

The meaning of this sutra is: Our sensory organs, i.e. eyes, ears, nose, tongue, skin are always attracted to external objects, for their nature tends towards objectivity. The moment there is an absence of their application towards the mundane sphere, they are automatically diverted inwards. The internalised citta gets dissolved into Aham, and Aham further into Mahat. This is called PRATYÁHÁRA yoga.

It can be explained elaborately like this: The propensities of human beings are naturally extroverted; humans are undergoing so many saḿskáras life after life, passing through weal and woe, pleasure and pain. By withdrawing the sensory organs from the objective world one cannot rid oneself of the mental bondages of action and reaction. So finally, by practising PRATYÁHÁRA mentally, the sádhaka, spiritual aspirant, can offer all the different colours of these different bondages at the lotus feet of the Cosmic Consciousness. The proper means to do this perfectly, with full attention and a fully concentrated mind is called; PRATYÁHÁRA SÁDHANÁ.

6. DHÁRAŃÁ

Dháraná is the concentration of the mind-stuff (Citta) in a particular point or region. When the physical body has achieved balance through the practice of ásanas there is proper hormone secretion, allowing control of emotions. The nervous system and mind have been stilled and calmed by the practice of Pránáyáma, and the activities of the sensory and motor organs are properly sublimated through Pratyáhára. The sádhaka (meditator) is then able to reach the higher stage of Dháraná, the sixth stage according to the Aśtáuṇga Yoga System.

The mental states experienced by the practitioner can be described in five stages. Before the mind can be completely and finally concentrated and absorbed in eternal Bliss, one has to be removed from other states of mind.

The first of these is kśipta state, where the mind is scattered and hankers after physical objects.

In the second state, called vikśipta, the mind is agitated and distracted. Here the mind enjoys the fruit of it's desire to some extent, but by being out of control it finally gets scattered without achieving it's goal.

The third state is called múrha, where the mind is static, dull and inert. The cover of static force brings the mind away from spirit.

The fourth state of mind is ekágra, when mind is focussed or concentrated in one point only. In this situation the mind cannot be pulled and pushed by mutative and static forces. One can easily achieve the desired object. So, when someone wants to succeed in life one has to achieve that ekágra state of mind.

The last state of mind is niruddha -when sádhaná, sádhaka and sádhya become one. Here there is no boundary between subject and object, when the mind, the intellect and the ego, with it's I feeling, merge, one gets dissolved in this state of mind. The sense of "own mind" is lost, the devotee becomes the machine and the Lord is the machine man.

7. DHYÁNA

"Every entity has its own movement. Nothing is stationary in this world. Everything moves. And I say, everything in this world is in a moving panorama, a passing show, a moving picture".

Everything is moving, passing by. In this changing phenomena and passing show we have to keep pace, we have to keep equipoise and equilibrium. It is like two trains travelling side by side together; as if we are each sitting in a different train, with the windows open, looking at each other and enjoying, laughing and talking together for hours with the same speed and momentum.

This is the Dhyána sádhaná – to have the mind adjust with His secret. Now, the subject of meditation (Dhyeya) is always busy with His creation. He has no time to sleep and to take rest. So, the devotee also must keep pace with that movement. One has to maintain the parallelism with the speed of His movement.

When the uninterrupted flow of divine Love is flowing as from a vessel of oil... pouring down incessantly, it is called "Taeladhárávat ekatánatá". If you observe a waterfall cascading down rhythmically from top to bottom with a continual flow, it appears to be a stationary line, as if someone drew a straight line, which is seen from far away as a thread. The reality is that this line is not stationary, there is in fact powerful dynamic movement taking place. This is the same state of mind one feels in Dhyána. The entitative flow of unit mind moves in the flow of the Cosmic mind. The sádhaka says, "In Your Dhyána, even if You move faster with tremendous flow and try Your best to be away from me, still I will keep holding You, and even if You don't want to be caught, I will not leave You.

" This is called "Taeladhárávat Ekatánatá".

The Cosmic Consciousness pervades each and every entity and object. The infinite emanation of the Cosmic Consciousness therefore naturally exists within and around the yogi or meditator. As He manifests Himself through us, we are beautiful and magnificent. When a spiritual practitioner becomes the proper medium, leaving all ego, senses, intellect and mind, he/she becomes a free channel of the Cosmic Consciousness. In this state, the spiritual practitioner experiences an uninterrupted flow of His divine love. In the midst of His Supreme universal love, the yogi becomes intoxicated with bliss and the love flows constantly. He is never alone. The force that guides the cosmologic order is also guiding the devotees towards the Supreme State. No words can explain that experience. Only the meditators can enjoy the state of Dhyána.

There is a fundamental difference between Dhyána and Dháraná. When the mind is given some boundary, confining it to a particular idea or entity, that is dháraná. Suppose, we keep our mind within a circle, within a boundary in some particular place and space and in no way do we allow our mind to wonder - that is called Dháraná.

And, what is Dhyána? Dhyána does not mean to put the mind in a figure. In dhyána the sádhaka runs after the Supreme Idea.

8. SAMÁDHI

It is the state in which a meditator, with his or her unit consciousness, becomes united with the cosmic consciousness and s/he loses their I-feeling or sense of separateness. In the Upaniśad it is mentioned:

"As a crystal of salt thrown into water dissolves and becomes one with water, so the state in which unity between one's 'I' consciousness and Supreme Consciousness is achieved, is called Samádhi".

The mind, operating in the sensory level, gets distracted with the influence of Máyá. That is the root cause of all worldly problems. In Samádhi, the mind is devoid of restlessness, 'I'ness, pleasure and pain. And if the mind is dissolved by constant ideation and channelisation of sensory desires, all love is directed towards the Supreme Being; one is fully attracted and absorbed in Him and experiences all bliss in Him.

In that state there are no objects, no passions, no aversions but there is ultimate satisfaction in the Supreme power of the Supreme happiness. So, Pátainjali explains:

"When the object of meditation engulfs the meditator, appearing as the subject, self-awareness is lost. This is Samádhi."

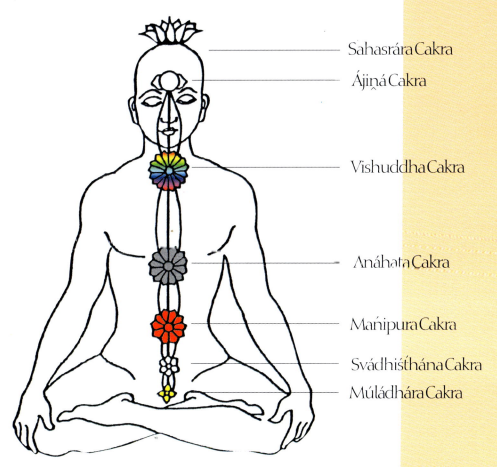

YOGA AND BIO-PSYCHOLOGY

A perfect psychology can only be expressed through a perfect biological structure. In the ladder of evolution, a human being comes into existence after a journey of millions of years. The human framework, the biological structure consists of a complex nervous system, a battery of hormones and an extensive lymphoid system to nourish and protect the nerve cells and the glands that secrete these hormones. The new science of biopsychology deals with the interaction between mental propensities, hormones and nerve cells and their effects on human behaviour.

In modern psychology, we study the mind by observing the behaviour, which is expressed externally. In yoga psychology, the mind is studied through introspective methods. The different techniques of meditation provide a method for the exercise of the inner mind, of the 'mental body' of a sádhaka. While doing yoga meditation, working with the body through ásanas and postures and concentrating the mind with constant attention, the meditator goes beyond the thoughts and reaches the level where s/he is 'lost in thought'. Where the devotee is beyond the awareness of 'body' and 'mind'.

As we use our bodies, we also use our minds. That part of ourselves, which observes our mind and mental functions, our thinking, feeling, willing and desiring, can learn to regulate these functions, control them, observe them and destroy them or more clearly which course of action may be best.

Our human growth through the process of biological evolution from protozoan to man is integrated with our psychological growth from childhood to adulthood. In order to discover and experience our wholeness as human beings, we will definitely need to tread the path of yoga. Our expansion through the five layers of the human mind will assist us in reaching the highest level of evolution.

All energy originates from the sun, endowing the elements of the planet such as air, light and water, with vitality in potential form. Human beings receive this energy mainly through the food we eat. After eating, these materials are transformed, passing through definite stages at which they can be utilized in the maintenance and development of our psycho-physical structure.

After the initial digestive process is complete, waste material is eliminated, and the remaining matter termed "Rasa" becomes the base material for the formation of blood.

The blood is a liquid tissue consisting of protein rich plasma, red and white blood cells. The essential nutrients that were contained in our food are refined, entering the blood in a form that can be specifically used by the body. The blood transports nutrients, oxygen and hormones to cells and serves as a mechanism for the removal of waste and toxins. The cells that comprise the connective tissue, nerve, muscle and bone of our physical structure are able to regenerate via the sustenance of the Rasa contained in blood.

The majority of cells in our body tissue are renewed every twenty-one days. Upon further refinement the Rasa becomes a more subtle matter called Vasa or Meda. With this Vasa the body can readily form the specialized cells of bone and bone marrow.

SHUKRA

Bone marrow is the site for formation of shukra. Shukra is the premier vital nourishing fluid of the human body. It is the cream of all we eat and drink, having passed through several stages of refinement within the body. For this reason, pure, wholesome food and drink is essential. Shukra exists in three stages, Lymph, Spermatozoa and Seminal fluid.

The human body contains about 50% more lymphatic fluid than blood. The function of lymph is to purify the blood and maintain the lustre and vitality of the body. Lymph has a critical role in the upkeep of the glands and the production of hormones, thereby having an enormous importance for our mental and physical well being.

The lymphatic system includes a network of capillaries that run side by side with the arteries. Lymphatic fluid passing through these vessels interacts with the blood, nourishing it and carrying away toxins and other debris.

Lymphatic fluid originating in the bone marrow becomes part of the blood plasma and can seep into the lymphatic vessels and into the interstitial spaces of tissue and organ cells. The lymph vessels carrying the proteinacious fluid interact with the blood nourishing it and carrying away toxins and other debris.

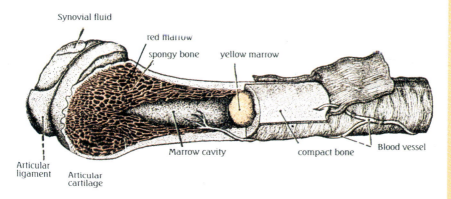

Diagram of the structure of long bones and joints

The immune function of the lymphatic system is observable at the microscopic level where lymphocytes are important elements. Lymph nodes lying along the course of the lymphatic vessels collect and degrade waste products and cellular debris from the tissues, eliminating toxins from the body.

In Yogic Practitioners, the major portion of the lymph remains in the body nourishing the brain and resulting in a higher intellectual standard.

THE MIND, YOGIC PRACTICE AND LYMPH

Lymph is an essential raw food for glands. Several glands and sub-glands in the human body are dependent upon lymph. There are many lymphatic glands in the body, which manufacture lymph. It is the initial hormone, and other glands use lymph to manufacture their respective hormones. Hormones are created when lymph comes in contact with an activated gland. By interacting with the glands it is transformed and enables the proper secretion of hormones.

The thoughts and emotions that predominate and determine our moods and mental states are largely influenced by presence of hormones in our bodies. The nourishment and balance of our glands and sub-glands with adequate lymph supply is therefore an important consideration for our physical and mental well-being.

Lymph is the vital food for the subtle glandular organs and also for the brain. Surplus lymph moves to the brain and provides food for the nerve cells in the cranium. For the proper development of innate qualities, such as clear intellect and subtle perception, an adequate amount of lymph is needed. The brain composition and function is strengthened by the proper supply of lymph.

In the male body after adequate supply of lymph has been provided to the brain, contact with the testes transforms this lymph into spermatozoa and seminal fluid. In females this excess becomes ova, and a certain proportion of lymph may also be used in the production of milk. In both sexes, excess lymph is discharged naturally and without harm.

A vegetarian diet is also congenial to the production of more lymph, as this vital fluid is produced more readily from foods, such as wheat grass and spinach, which contain high levels of chlorophyll.

The nature of our thoughts influences the formation of lymph and its availability. For example, impure thoughts or environment can cause an excessive formation of spermatozoa from lymph, reducing the amount available for the brain. Certain psychological or physico-psychic factors may act as positive and negative triggers in the manufacture of lymph. A good environment – both physical and psychic, such as a pure forest or beach – acts as a positive influence.

Positive psychic and physical environments are positive triggers, and negative psychic and physical environments, such as polluted commercial centres or eating while under the influence of anger or stress, are negative triggers.

If food is sentient, but the environment is negative, for example fresh fruit consumed in a polluted subway, such a condition is detrimental and the result may be that, lymph is not utilised by the glands in the optimum way for our overall psycho-physical well being. In this way we can begin to understand the scientific relationship, described by yoga, that exists between our environment, our thinking and our physical health.

"The main purpose of human beings coming here to this earth is to do Sádhaná. By Spiritual Sádhaná, (Yogic Practice) you may bring about certain changes in your nervous system, nerve cells and nerve fibres, control the secretions of the hormones from different glands and sub-glands, and become elevated superhuman and go beyond the periphery of the common psychology".

SHRII SHRII ÁNANDAMÚRTII

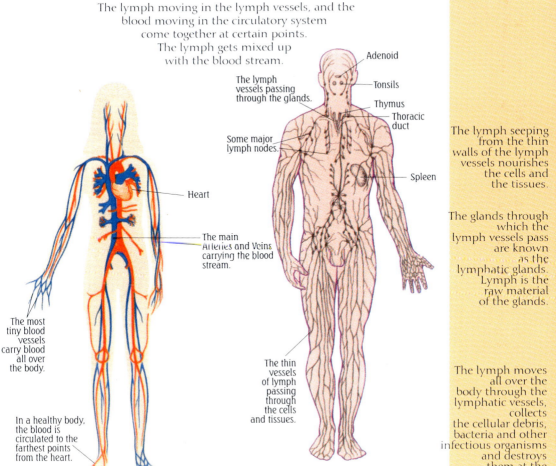

39

GLANDS, SUB-GLANDS AND ENDOCRINE SYSTEM

The human body is a biological machine. Improper secretion of a gland or series of glands will bring the machine under different impulses, resulting in changes in one's physical and psychic expression. Millions of specialized secretory tissues exist in the human body.

There are two major types of glands: endocrine and exocrine. Exocrine glands secrete their contents into ducts that carry them to their site of action. The specialized endocrine glands such as the Pituitary, the Thyroid and the Gonads produce small to tremendous effects by directly secreting hormones into the bloodstream. From here the chemical messengers reach their targets and produce changes in both the body and mind. Functions such as body temperature, energy level, adrenaline, sexuality, growth, etc. are regulated by endocrine gland secretion.

Levels of hormone secretion have a profound effect on our mental state. An example is the hormone adrenaline, secreted from the adrenal glands at times of high stress or fear. It produces the "fight or flight" physico-psychic response resulting in mental alertness, dilated pupils, increase of the blood flow to the muscles and a negation of appetite and digestion processes. Studies have shown that in response to adrenaline there is a notable fall in the ability to recall information stored in the long-term memory. This is consistent with the need to think in the moment in a dangerous situation. Individuals with a hyper-secretion of adrenaline regularly experience chronic stress, the result of a protracted alert state created by the hormone, including inability to remember important information when needed. Similarly, hyperactivity in the thyroid gland resulting in excess thyroxin hormone results in nervousness, weight loss, and causing dramatic changes in the metabolic rate.

The main endocrine glands:
1 - Pineal
2 - Pituitary
3 - Parathyroid
4 - Thyroid
5 - Thymus
6 - Adrenal
7 - Gonads
   Ovaries in the female
   and testes in the male

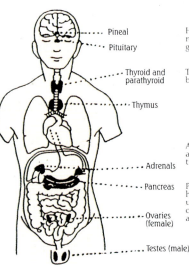

Pineal
Pituitary
Thyroid and parathyroid
Thymus
Adrenals
Pancreas
Ovaries (female)
Testes (male)

Hypothalamus regulates, controls the work of other glands in the body.

Thyroid and parathyroid glands, balance the basal metabolic rate.

Adrenal glands produce adrenaline as a response to the stress of the mind.

Pancreas produces insulin hormone promoting the uptake of glucose by body cells and balances the amount of glucose in blood.

These examples illustrate the direct relationship between hormone secretion, physiological homeostasis and the emotions experienced by human beings. The endocrine glands influence the cells, and together with the glands and the nervous system, the mind is also influenced. Yogic science details the practical way by which, through proper physical and mental adjustment and sentient feeling, the mind goes through the channel of wholeness.

Ásanas are calm, quiet and easy postures held with proper breathing. They are postures that will help to achieve physical and mental well-being. With regular practice, ásanas keep the body healthy and cure many diseases. This is acheived by correcting the defective glands and balancing hormonal secretions.

In this way, ásanas may have a profound effect on the glands and sub-glands. All ásanas have either a pressurizing or depressurizing effect on the glands and sub-glands. For example, sarváuṇgásana (see page 91) has a pressurizing effect on the thyroid. The secretions of the glands and sub-glands of the Vishuddha Cakra and the propensities associated with them will become more balanced if this ásana is practised regularly. If someone has improper thyroxine hormone secretion, it means his or her Vishuddha Cakra is imbalanced. Through the regular practice of sarváuṇgásana, the secretion of the hormone may be controlled. Matsyásana may have a depressurizing effect on the Cakra, and if these ásanas are performed regularly the glands and sub-glands associated with the cakra will become balanced. By practicing ásanas regularly one can control the propensities and either increase or decrease their activity.

THE MAJOR GLANDS AND SUB-GLANDS

PINEAL GLAND

The Pineal Gland is a tiny mushroom shaped gland weighing about 100mg located directly in the middle of the brain. The importance of the Pineal Gland has not yet been fully understood by modern science. In the 17 Century, Rene Descartes termed the gland "the seat of the rational soul". Yogic Science explains the critical role of the Pineal Gland as the master controlling gland of the human body, ultimately controlling all the glands. More recent research has begun to reveal the far-reaching influences of the Pineal Gland.

Studies have found that the pineal gland secretes the hormones Melatonin and Serotonin. Melatonin is the only hormone to have been isolated. These two hormones affect the mind and body directly or indirectly through activation of the glands below. The pineal gland is extremely sensitive to light. During the darkness of night the amount of melatonin is very high and the amount of serotonin is very low. This produces a very relaxed state of mind so that the person can easily fall asleep. During the day time the opposite occurs – low melatonin and high serotonin produce a more restless state of activity.

Modern experimentation suggests that melatonin is involved in maintaining vitality and life, increasing the lifespan by 20% in experimental animals; also reducing cosmetic effects and incidence of illness associated with aging. A relationship with the immune system has also been found suggesting the hormone may increase antibody (specialized immune cell) production.

If the production of serotonin is gradually decreased, a person may experience more peaceful states, eventually entering states of higher awareness. The person may experience deep peace or blissful feelings.

The pineal gland seems to work in the opposite direction to most of the other glands in the body. When these glands are at the peak of their function, the pineal gland seems to be dormant, and when they are resting, the pineal gland is awake.

Other glands are driving us to "do things", while the pineal gland is restraining them. There is an inverse relationship between the pineal gland and the endocrine glands – increased stimulation of the endocrine glands leads to a decreased stimulation of the pineal gland and vice versa. If we maintain a high level of stimulation of the endocrine glands it becomes harmful to the body – for example, in the case of an overactive thyroid gland. Therefore the pineal gland must maintain a balance in the body where conscious activity can be performed and the mind can also be internalised. With Yogic practice, the physical expression of the inverse relationship is diminished, allowing a more balanced state to be maintained.

PITUITARY GLAND

Modern science considers the Pituitary to be the master-controlling gland. The pituitary however, receives directions from the Hypothalamus, engaging in an array of actions based on these signals. Some hormones secreted by the Hypothalamus trigger, important processes include ACTH – adrenocorticotrophic hormone that stimulates the adrenal gland; TSH – thyroid stimulating hormone which prompts the production of thyroxin; (growth, development and temperature control are all stimulated by pituitary hormones). Pituitary hormones also influence the movement of the bowels, kidney function and the vascular tone of the blood vessels.

Yogic Science explains the important role of the pituitary. Where spiritual progress is manifested through the activity of the pineal gland, psycho-spiritual progress takes place through the pituitary gland. It means that the effects of our intuitive expansion are mediated by the pituitary gland. The conscious, subconscious and unconscious portions of the mind are controlled via this point.

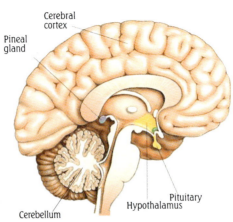

Cerebral cortex Pituitary and Pineal glands

THYROID AND PARATHYROID GLANDS

The Thyroid gland is situated in the neck with lobes spanning both the sides of the larynx. It produces the hormones Thyroxine and Calcitonin. Calcitonin decreases calcium levels in the blood and the secretions of the Parathyroid gland increase blood calcium levels, and regulate phosphorus metabolism. The level of Thyroxine secretion has serious effects on the body-mind. Over secretion can result in an increased metabolic rate. Cellular respiration is accelerated and even at rest the rate of consumed oxygen increases, as does the heart rate, which results in an increase in blood pressure.

Symptoms are extreme worry; nervousness; insomnia, paranoia and weight loss. In this over-activated state the nervous system becomes exhausted, the eyeballs may protrude.

Under-secretion of thyroxine displays symptoms of low heart rate, mental dullness, dry skin, intolerance to cold, lack of energy, lethargy and tiredness. This, in infancy affects the development of the brain cells and may lead to permanent mental deficiency and dwarfism.

The pea-sized parathyroid glands are located behind or within the thyroid gland. They maintain blood calcium levels by increasing calcium absorption in the intestine. These glands work as a fine-tuning mechanism, for regulating blood calcium. If blood calcium increases, this increase acts directly on the gland to inhibit the secretion of the hormone. This is called "Negative feed back system". The best way to regulate the hormone secretions is to follow the natural path of yoga ásanas.

According to Yogic science, the thyroid and parathyroid glands are closely related to mental development and intellectual elevation. Normal body processes and normal thinking require the exact amount of thyroid hormones to be secreted at all times. For example, the over-secretion of thyroid hormones may cause a person to become irrational and of quarrelsome nature. Vanity, too, may develop if there is under secretion of the parathyroid gland.

THYMUS GLAND

The Thymus is a bi-lobular lymphatic gland located behind the sternum bone of the chest. This gland is most active during childhood and then shrinks to a quarter of it's original size at the time of puberty. The gland's main role is in the immune function of the body, producing T-lymphocyte cells that help defend the body against infection. Other functions of the thymus are not known. The Solar Plexus region of the body where the thymus is positioned is associated with the reception and transmission of subtle energy. In this way the reception of positive subtle energy directly influences our immune capacity. Similarly, negative energy accepted by this region weakens our immune response.

ADRENAL GLANDS

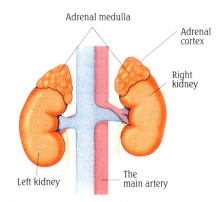

These glands are located just above each kidney (hence ad-renal). The outer cortex produces corticosteroids that regulate blood concentration and influence metabolic rate. Their release increases during periods of stress associated with events such as facing new situations or any exciting condition. The adrenal cortex also produces a small amount of male sex hormones in both men and women. These hormones may consequently cause the growth of facial hair and masculine characteristics in women. Bearded ladies are victims of such hormonal disorders.

The inner medulla produces adrenaline, which is associated with the sudden bursts of energy in response to danger or stress (the fight or flight response mentioned above). In primitive times people would utilize the energy produced by this response to fight against danger or run away from trouble. In modern society this stress response cannot be discharged or dissipated so easily. As a result, the concentration of glucose in the blood stream is increased, respiration is stimulated and blood pressure is increased. It is for this reason that there has been a growing trend towards stress related diseases such as high blood pressure, heart disease, peptic ulcers etc. Yogic practices and breathe related exercices not only help to balance the secretions of these hormones, but they also allow the body to experience deep relaxation, dissipating the impact of the accumulated stress on the body.

THE GONADS

The name Gonads refers collectively to the glands controlling the sexual function – the testes and ovaries. These glands secrete Androgens (male sex hormones) and Estrogens (female sex hormones). These hormones regulate the development of the body throughout the passage to adulthood, eg. puberty and growth, and later menopause. They also have a central role in the psycho-physical expression of the individual. For example Androgens increase the muscular mass and may also induce aggressive behaviour. Estrogens increase the proportion of fatty tissue in the body.

According to Yogic science, if there is over-activity of the sexual glands, a sense of responsibility and dutifulness develops during youth. In between the ages of 15 and 18 this hyper-secretion of sex hormones inspires the deep urge to "do something great" as well as the physical changes we normally associate with sexual maturity and maintaining sexual characteristics in both males and females.

Both the testes and ovaries serve two functions:
    *The production of reproductive cells.
    *The production of accessory hormones such as testosterone, prostate…

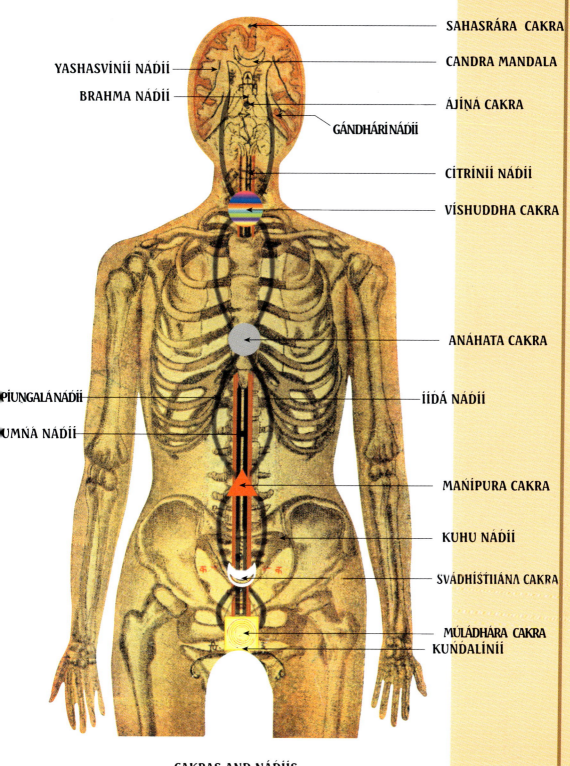

CAKRAS AND NÁDIIS
ENERGY CENTERS AND ENERGY CHANNELS

YOGA PHYSIOLOGY

Modern science is uncovering more and more evidence, which is enlightening our understanding of the interrelationship between our thoughts, perceptions and the physiology and pathology of what we understand as our physical bodies. The ancient science of Yoga is based on the understanding that we are, in fact, a completely integrated mind-body machine.

Yogic exercises and practices are a scientific method by which we can attain perfect physical health. By developing a fit, healthy body with balanced hormone secretions, healthy internal organs, a robust and toned musculo-skeletal system and good circulation, our mind can be free from the physical sphere and move towards higher pursuits. Every aspect of the human being's physiology is benefited from yoga practice. It has a particularly significant influence on the glandular and lymphatic systems, discussed below. In many instances, yogic science describes subtle mind-body physiology at a deeper level than has as yet been documented in modern research. We can understand these relationships as practitioners of yoga had for thousands of years, through our own practical experimentation, observing the effect on our mind and body when we practise yoga. In the following pages I have described in some detail the important physiological effects of yoga practice where appropriate with reference to the contemporary scientific terminology and theory.

THE MUSCULAR SYSTEM

Muscle is a specialized tissue that can contract or shorten in response to the impulses from the central nervous system. There are three types of muscle comprising nearly forty percent of our body weight. Skeletal muscles control body movement and maintain body posture. Smooth muscle is found in the walls of our internal organs and as the name suggests, cardiac muscles form the walls of the heart.

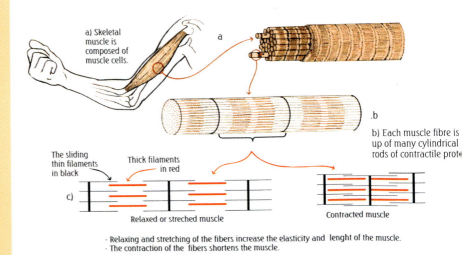

c) Electron micrograph and the diagram of a myofibril. The thick filaments in red; the thin filaments in black. Contraction, relaxation and stretching of the muscle involves the sliding of the thin filament between the thick ones by opening a free zone where blood is easily carried. So a stretched and relaxed muscle receives more oxygen than a contracted one.

a) Skeletal muscle is composed of muscle cells.

b) Each muscle fibre is up of many cylindrical rods of contractile prot

The sliding thin filaments in black

Thick filaments in red

Relaxed or streched muscle

Contracted muscle

- Relaxing and stretching of the fibers increase the elasticity and lenght of the muscle.
- The contraction of the fibers shortens the muscle.

Typically, physical exercise works the skeletal muscles by repetitive movements of contraction and expansion. These may be rapidly repeated and result in the building up of the muscles that are being used. Yoga exercises (ásanas) in contrast, involve slow contraction of the muscles through gradual movement. During ásana practice, normal breathing is sufficient to maintain the necessary oxygen that the body requires, so there is no accumulation of toxic by-products such as lactic acid in the body. In addition, as ásanas are practiced in a calm and quiet way, there is no adrenaline hormone released in the body. This allows the body and mind to remain in a tranquil state without fatigue.

Where regular physical exercise works predominantly on selected groups of skeletal muscles, Yoga ásanas exercise all the muscles of different parts of the body. They also massage the smooth muscles of internal organs such as the stomach and intestine. This gentle pressure influences the internal organs themselves, stretching them and improving their vitality and function through improved blood circulation.

THE CIRCULATORY SYSTEM

Heart and blood pressure related illnesses are a major cause of disease throughout the world today. Efficient circulation depends on a healthy heart and supple and unobstructed blood vessels, from the major arteries and veins to the tiny capillaries. Disease typically occurs when obstructions such as fatty deposits in the arteries, inelastic artery walls or poorly functioning valves in the blood vessels inhibit the flow of blood. This places increased strain on the heart, as it has to work harder to deliver blood to the different regions of the body. We commonly hear of 'heart attacks' and 'angina' resulting from inadequate supply of blood to the heart, high blood pressure - as a result of increased resistance in the vessels, and stroke - the result of blockage of blood flowing to the brain. Diseases in other organs also arise due to inadequate blood supply and the accumulation of toxins.

Yogic ásanas are isometric exercises, which means they rely on holding muscle tension for a short period of time. This improves cardiovascular fitness and blood circulation. Research shows that regular yoga practice may help to normalize blood pressure. The twisting and stretching movements performed during yoga ásanas stretch the blood vessels, maintaining their elasticity and promoting the clearance of toxic accumulations and fatty deposits that obstruct blood flow. In addition, the valves that ensure correct flow of blood on its way back to the heart get the chance to rest and revitalize. During yoga postures such as sarváungásana, the inverted position enables free blood flow by gravitational force back to the heart. The inverted postures also permit complete clearance of blood and toxins that may have pooled in veins of the feet and legs.

In this way Yogic practice can allow us to maintain good health and longevity of life through a sound circulatory system that efficiently transports oxygen and nutrients to the various organs, boosting our vital energy and allowing us to stay active, alert and energetic longer.

THE SPINAL COLUMN

Nerves from the brain and spine are connected with every tissue in the body and therefore the health of the entire body is influenced by the health of the brain and spine. The vertebral column consists of 33 vertebrae supporting the head and trunk. Cartilage discs between the pairs of vertebrae allow for limited individual and wide ranging collective flexibility. This enables the range of body movement we are familiar with.

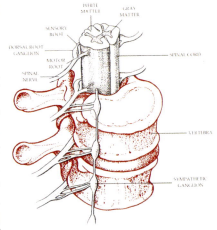

The paravertebral muscles surrounding the spine maintain balance when the spine is not held in its proper posture. Holding poor posture for extended periods of time, places strain upon these muscles and leads to chronic back pain. Over a prolonged time period this leads to stiffening of the vertebrae due to shortening in the tendons and ligaments. This compresses the spinal nerves causing pain and discomfort and reducing the range of movement one can easily perform.

A segment of the human spinal cord. Each spinal nerve divides into two fiber bundles. The sensory and motor roots. Sympathetic ganglia are part of autonomic nervous system. (see details next page)

The ancient yogis fully understood the importance of the spinal column in maintaining excellent health. They knew that keeping the spine supple by yoga ásanas meant there would be much less chance of spinal stiffening. Many ásanas directly stretch the ligaments and tendons allowing the practitioner to maintain excellent posture and the full array of movement. In this way the yogic practice prevents the degeneration of the spine that develop in a large proportion of people after about age thirty.

Orthopedic medical specialists recommend yoga practice as a means to maintain a healthy spinal column. Notably, yoga ásanas are prescribed for the treatment and prevention of osteoporosis, a degenerative condition of the bones of the vertebra, affecting two out of three women in developed nations and one out of three men.

HEALTHY JOINTS

The bones of the human body are connected with each other at their ends by ligaments at the joints. Joints are under constant stress as they absorb shock associated with physical movement and support the weight force of the entire body. Studies have concluded that a major cause of arthritis (inflammation of the joints) is the accumulation of toxic deposits such as calcium and uric acid. The stretching of the joints in ásanas causes the secretion of a lubricant called synovial fluid. This slow stretching combine with the presence of adequate synovial fluid, removes toxins and allows the joints to maintain their full function and health.

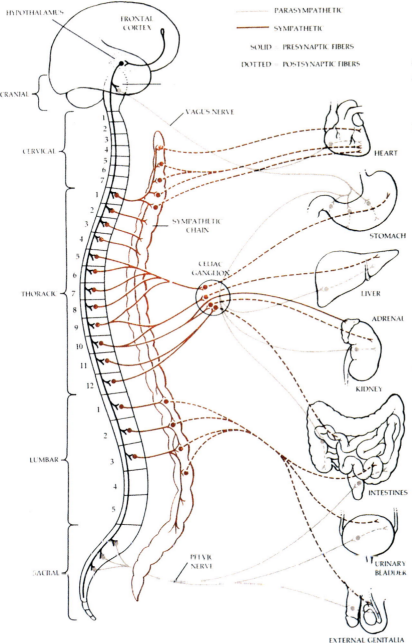

Divisions of the Autonomic Nervous System, consisting of the sympathetic fibres of the parasympathetic sytem. Internal organs are innervated by both systems. The Sympathetic system produces the effect of exciting organs "fight or flight" reactions. The Parasympathetic system stimulates more tranquil functions, such as digestion. Here you can follow the connection of the nerves.

The different organs of the body are connected to the central nervous system located in the vertebrae. Any disturbance in the vertebrae such as dislocation etc. causes ailments in the central nervous system and affects the concerned internal organs due to the defect in the system as a whole.

The habit of keeping the body straight has a major effect on our health. Regular performance of Yoga ásanas helps us to create healthy backbones by stretching, relaxing and strengthening the backbone muscles. Our central nervous system and internal organs will be positively effected.

DIVISIONS	CNS CONNECTIONS	POINT OF SYNAPSE	EFFECTS
Sympathetic	Thoracic and lumbar regions of spinal cord	Ganglia near spinal cord	Helps organism to cope with external environment
Para-sympathetic	Brain stem and sacral (tail) area of spinal cord	Ganglia near target organ	Supports restorative, resting body functions

INTRODUCTION TO ÁSANAS

*"Just as diseased body
organs can be restored to normal by
administering medicines internally or externally,
they can also be healed, more safely and more perfectly,
with the help of Yaogika Ásanas…"*
— Shrii Shrii Ánandamúrti

Ásanas are widely known as the main practice of Hatha Yoga. They form a major component of Aśtáunga Yoga, which is encompassed by Rájádhirája Yoga. Yoga meditation can only be performed by those who are physically healthy and have sound mental balance. Hence, ásanas or yoga postures are of profound importance for the sincere yoga practitioner.

The first two components of Aśtáunga Yoga are Yama and Niyama, which help the practitioner to form a pure mental and physical base. The practice of yoga ásanas creates balance in the body's glandular system. Of the thousands of ásanas in existence, most cannot be learned in one lifetime and anyway this endeavour is not necessary for one to achieve complete physico-psychic balance.

The selected ásanas described in this chapter are beneficial for both the body and mind.

These ásanas were chosen for their wide ranging benefits to health and intuitional practice. They are presented in a systematic way, beginning with simple postures and building up to the more difficult ones.

One does not need to perform all the postures every time one practices, three or four are enough if done precisely according to the guidance. Of course, if one has the time to practise longer it will certainly be beneficial. In this section of the book the benefits derived from the ásanas are clearly detailed with special reference to their curative capacity. One ásana can be very helpful for several ailments and likewise, for one type of ailment there may be many ásanas.

Perhaps more important than their curative effect, the regular practice of yoga exercises acts as a preventive measure against sickness and disease. By strengthening the immune system and aiding in the break-down and expulsion of toxins we maintain good health. The endocrine effect of performing ásanas balances our emotional state helping to keep the mind flowing freely and positively, influencing our overall wellbeing. A yogic lifestyle thus allows the maintenance of excellent health by preventing illness from occurring, as well as through its curative capacity.

Several studies have described the lower stress levels observed in yogic practitioners. Using yogic methods, we avoid the risk of side-effects associated with chemical or toxic treatments, the general worry and anxiety related to disease as well as unnecessary medical expenses. Yogic practices represent a completely natural system for sustaining good health.

padmásana

1

In Saṁskṛta padma means lotus and ásana means position comfortably held.

BENEFITS

Wherever possible one should sit straight with an erect spine.

This helps concentration, improves the memory and as a result strengthens one's will power.

If this posture is maintained from childhood then one retains youthfulness

Good for mental work especially in old age

This posture assists the flow of the body's vital fluids.

With regular practice one obtains a feeling of peace and tranquillity.

It treats abdominal diseases, as well as female disorders connected to the reproductive system.

The Lotus posture helps in Japa, dhyána and sádhaná,(types of spiritual practices), by stimulating the endocrine glands.

It helps those suffering from asthma, insomnia and hysteria

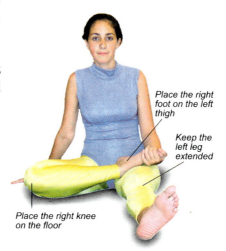

Place the right foot on the left thigh
Keep the left leg extended
Place the right knee on the floor

STEP 1

In order to practice the lotus posture first warm up the legs using the butterfly technique; that is touch the soles of the feet together then interlocking the fingers around the toes gently pull the feet towards the body and, continuing to hold the toes, flap the knees up and down like the wings of a butterfly. This motion will loosen the knots in the thighs making padmásana much easier. After warming up extend the left leg placing the right foot on the left thigh (see photo), gently lifting and lowering the right knee until it comes to rest on the ground.

STEP 2

Bending the left knee grasp the left ankle and gradually pull it towards the body, lifting and placing it above the right calf.

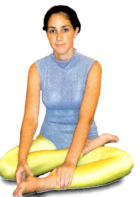

Grasp the left leg and place it on the top of the other leg

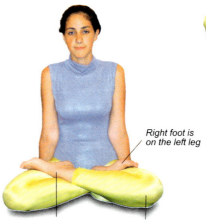

Right foot is on the left leg
Left foot is on the top of the right leg
Left knee is touching to floor

STEP 3

While placing the left foot on the right leg take care the right foot does not slip otherwise a loss of balance will occur. Try to rest the knees on the ground.

LOTUS POSTURE

STEP 4
This is the full lotus, the best posture for meditation and concentration. Interlocking the fingers rest the hands on the leg. Keep the eyes closed and let the breath flow freely.
For deeper learning seek guidance from a yoga and meditation instructor.

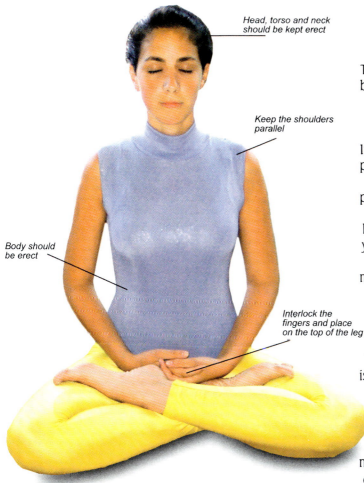

Head, torso and neck should be kept erect

Keep the shoulders parallel

Body should be erect

Interlock the fingers and place on the top of the leg

This ásana is concerned with the lower two cakras so it helps fight impotency in both males and females.

It is helpful for those suffering from psychic imbalance, especially depression.

Whilst sitting erectly in meditation the lotus posture makes the spinal cord ready to receive the kuńdalinii force when it rises. Because the spine is held erect, it allows the energy to rise up the spinal column.

This posture brings harmony between the body and mind, which can lead one to focus on divinity.

If one is not able to sit in lotus posture do not be discouraged but rather continue to persevere and eventually one will feel the tremendous benefits of this ásana. Teach your children this posture so that from an early age they may be able to benefit in their studies, relationships and other aspects of their everyday lives.

Excepting Shavásana, there is no other ásana (posture) by which body can be kept completely relaxed in erect position. This Padmásana is the only ásana, next to Shavásana where one can feel complete rest, calm and quiet provided one performs it sitting fully in a straight position.

2

viirásana

In Saṁskṛta the meaning of viira is bravery.

Pointing the toes backward sit on the heels keeping the knees together. Press the wrists on the top of the thighs keeping the arms straight and fingers pointing upwards. The back should be kept straight and eyes half closed and concentrated on the tip of the nose.

BENEFITS

This posture is considered the best for developing concentration and memory power.

When someone feels disturbed and the mind is scattered, or feelings of dullness and inertia arise, then one should sit in this ásana and look at the tip of the nose.

Keeping the eyes open and focussing the gaze at a particular point of one's body is part of the Trátak technique*. It is best to concentrate the gaze above the Vishuddha cakra.

The brave posture possesses the quality to help one to discover the answers to unsolved problems.

If Viirásana is practised from childhood then one attains the power of concentration very easily. The nature of the mind is to run uncontrollably from one thought to another, from one desire to the next. This posture helps to tame this nature, giving one the capacity to check the flow of thought, so that one can act in a calm and effective manner.

If the brave posture is perfected one will develop a sharp intellect and concentrated intuition. When this intellect is goaded towards intuitional practise one can achieve one pointedness (Agrá Buddhi) very easily.

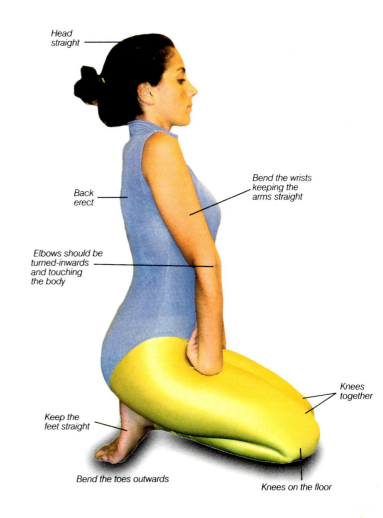

Head straight

Back erect

Bend the wrists keeping the arms straight

Elbows should be turned-inwards and touching the body

Keep the feet straight

Knees together

Bend the toes outwards

Knees on the floor

If you are keen to develop your yoga practise and meditation technique viirásana is greatly beneficial.

* Trátak technique: Trátak yoga is controlling the ocular vision. It may lead to some supernatural vision.

BRAVE POSTURE

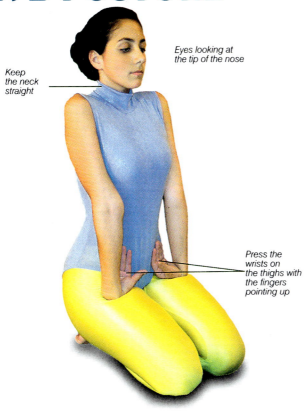

Keep the neck straight

Eyes looking at the tip of the nose

Press the wrists on the thighs with the fingers pointing up

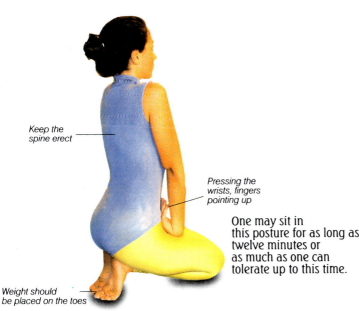

Keep the spine erect

Pressing the wrists, fingers pointing up

Weight should be placed on the toes

One may sit in this posture for as long as twelve minutes or as much as one can tolerate up to this time.

Fear is one of man's worst enemies, having the power to disable an individual and thereby halt their progress. This ásana endows the practitioner with bravery and ability to overcome fear and march ahead in life with courage and confidence.

By nature a human being possesses animal instincts such as eating, sleeping, reproduction. The brave ásana gives one the ability to overcome the complexes associated with these animal instincts and by gaining a certain level of control one can progress towards a higher level of existence.

Viirásana has a tremendously positive effect with respect to meditation and yoga, concentration and self development. One should perform this posture for at least twelve minutes (or as much as one can do).

This posture helps the practitioner to attain a high level of comprehension, so that one can understand and learn very quickly.

Fixing the gaze at a particular point helps to massage the optical nerves in the eyes, and along with regular eye exercises can cure many eye disorders.

The brave posture is a quick and effective cure for many stomach disorders. After eating it is good to formulate the habit of sitting in Brave posture for some time (preferably no less than twelve minutes) and then lying on the left side. This habit aids the body's digestive process.

yogamudrá

3 BENEFITS

Yogamudrá is an easy, yet highly effective posture and is prescribed as one of the essential ásanas for women. It works on many different parts of the body and is especially beneficial for eliminating fat, making the body strong and increasing will power.

Because of its ease this ásana is recommended for those who have not practised yoga in their youth. For middle-aged beginners it is advisable to start their yoga routine with this ásana.

This posture has a revitalising effect on the spleen, liver and heart and when performed properly and regularly, has the power to cure many ailments in these organs.

To get maximum benefit from yogamudrá one must focus one's attention on the breath, imagining that the cells of the body are being revitalised with every inhalation and that all the bodies toxins are being swept away while breathing out.

STEP 1

Sit straight and erect and concentrating on your breathing relax the body. Bringing both hands behind the back grasp the left wrist with the right hand.

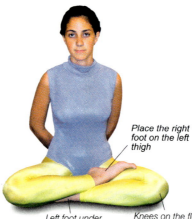

Place the right foot on the left thigh

Left foot under the right leg

Knees on the floor

If one cannot sit in half lotus one may sit cross-legged in any other comfortable position.

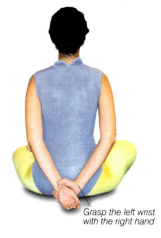

Grasp the left wrist with the right hand

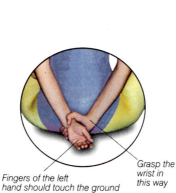

Fingers of the left hand should touch the ground

Grasp the wrist in this way

YOGA POSTURE

Regular practice keeps the spine flexible allowing the subtle energies to flow smoothly through the body so one will not suffer from any unnecessary tiredness, but rather enjoy an energetic youthfulness.

This posture is an aid for meditation and other introversive activities, allowing the erect posture to be maintained along with sustained concentration.

STEP 2

Exhaling slowly lower the forehead and nose trying to bring them in contact with the floor.
Maintain this ásana for eight seconds with breath fully exhaled.

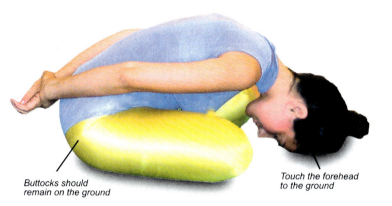

Buttocks should remain on the ground

Touch the forehead to the ground

Yogamudrá prepares the body for lotus posture, so if one has any difficulty performing padmásana one can make it a habit to sit erectly and practise this mudrá.

If one has free time one can start their routine of ásanas with yogamudrá. Alternatively, if for example, one is short of time it is better to start with the cobra.

STEP 3

Slowly inhale and raise the body upright to the sitting position.
Repeat eight times.

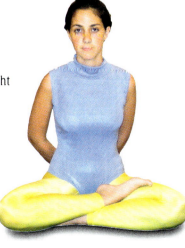

In the beginning one may not be able to touch the forehead to the floor but still one should make the effort gently pushing the body a little further while exhaling

4

diirgha praṋáma

In Saṁskrta diirgha praṋáma means long bowing posture

BENEFITS

Especially beneficial for women, the long bowing posture possesses all the benefits of yogamudrá and along with cobra is one of the three basic ásanas prescribed for females.

It is beneficial for curing many women's disorders, especially in relation to menstruation problems. Please note, it should not be performed during pregnancy.

This posture strengthens the abdominal muscles making the nerves and veins of the stomach strong. It is particularly good for relieving constipation, loosening the bloated stomach and releasing gas.

It helps one to lose excess weight and has a revitalising effect on the pancreas giving a fresh burst of life and vitality.

It benefits the lower three cakras, the solid, liquid and gaseous factors, allowing proper hormone secretion in those glands and thus enabling a balance between the mind and body, allowing the practitioner to enjoy a deeper rest.

This ásana when performed properly has the power to alleviate breathing disorders.

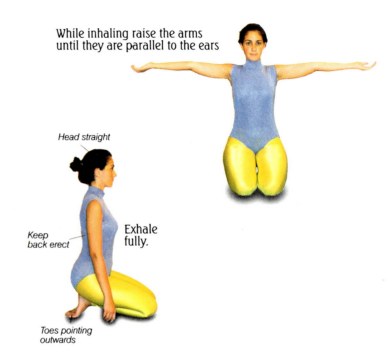

While inhaling raise the arms until they are parallel to the ears

Head straight

Keep back erect

Exhale fully.

Toes pointing outwards

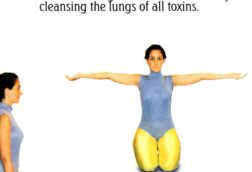

While lowering the arms exhale slowly, cleansing the lungs of all toxins.

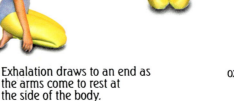

Exhalation draws to an end as the arms come to rest at the side of the body.

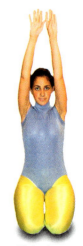

Fill the lungs with oxygen and stretch the arms high above the head.

LONG BOWING POSTURE

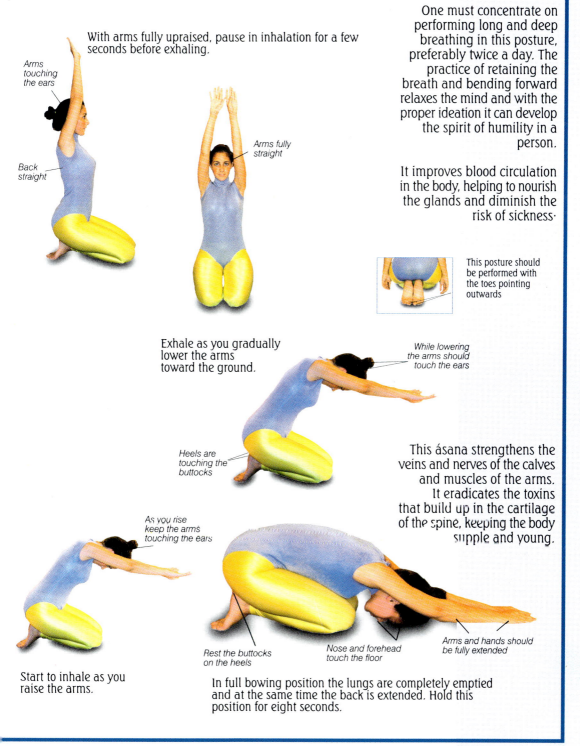

With arms fully upraised, pause in inhalation for a few seconds before exhaling.

Arms touching the ears

Back straight

Arms fully straight

One must concentrate on performing long and deep breathing in this posture, preferably twice a day. The practice of retaining the breath and bending forward relaxes the mind and with the proper ideation it can develop the spirit of humility in a person.

It improves blood circulation in the body, helping to nourish the glands and diminish the risk of sickness.

This posture should be performed with the toes pointing outwards

Exhale as you gradually lower the arms toward the ground.

While lowering the arms should touch the ears

Heels are touching the buttocks

This ásana strengthens the veins and nerves of the calves and muscles of the arms. It eradicates the toxins that build up in the cartilage of the spine, keeping the body supple and young.

As you rise keep the arms touching the ears

Rest the buttocks on the heels

Nose and forehead touch the floor

Arms and hands should be fully extended

Start to inhale as you raise the arms.

In full bowing position the lungs are completely emptied and at the same time the back is extended. Hold this position for eight seconds.

5 bhújauṅgásana

In Saṁskṛta bhújauṅga means snake yet this ásana is commonly known in English as the cobra, because little by little as you raise your head, shoulders and back, it resembles the posture of the poisonous cobra.

BENEFITS

The cobra posture has a therapeutic effect on the spine, removing pain one may have in that region. When practised frequently it has the power to revitalise the whole spinal column from neck to coccyx

It also fortifies the nerves and veins of the stomach and back and by exerting pressure on the abdomen it cures constipation along with other abdominal disorders.

The cobra beautifies the upper body by stretching, toning and shaping the chest, shoulders, arms and neck as well as reducing fat around the waist.

This ásana has the power to alleviate many common women's diseases, especially menstrual disorders, helping to revitalise the ovaries and support the uterus, easing the birth process.

It affects the Vishuddha and Ájiṅá cakras

Practising this ásana develops one's breathing capability, as one learns how to take slow and deep breaths filling the lungs entirely, thus enabling a greater intake of oxygen and a better circulation of the blood. At the same time practising to exhale fully rids the body of many toxins that in turn acts as a preventative measure against disease.

STEP 1
Lie down flat on the stomach with the elbows bent and palms parallel to the neck. Exhale fully.

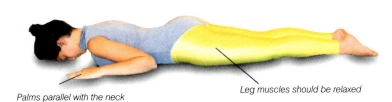

Palms parallel with the neck *Leg muscles should be relaxed*

STEP 2
Inhaling, gradually raise the head and shoulders and turn the eyes upwards. Keep the forearms firmly on the floor and hold for eight seconds.

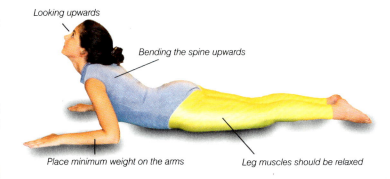

Looking upwards *Bending the spine upwards*
Place minimum weight on the arms *Leg muscles should be relaxed*

In the beginning practise this posture four to eight times.

Prevents the deformation and deterioration of the spine.

COBRA POSTURE

STEP 3
Repeat step 1. Inhaling, raise the head and shoulders, this time straightening the arms and further extending the head backwards. Hold for eight seconds and repeat four to eight times.

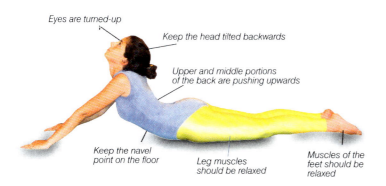

STEP 4
Repeat step 1. After fully exhaling, breathe in and raise the body up to the navel point, at the same time turning your gaze upwards. Try to gain maximum lift in the body.

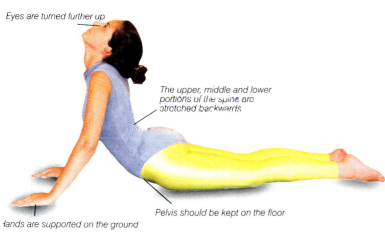

Retaining the breath this position should be held for eight seconds. Gradually lower the body and at the same time breathe out.

The cobra is prescribed for all sorts of back and neck pain.

The cobra posture prevents nose bleeds caused by temperature changes, as well as assisting to increase the heat in the body.

If performed correctly this ásana can greatly improve the flexibility of the spinal cord. As a result one slows down the decay of the spine and thus can remain youthful and active even in old age.

If the cobra is adopted early on in life, or if it is practised strictly with the proper breathing technique, it is the best cure against the build up of toxins in the body. By breaking down the body's toxins it prevents unnecessary physical disorders and thus mental suffering. For example extreme calcification is responsible for many ailments, including headaches and migraines, stiff joints and rheumatism.

In this modern age of speed and tension, where people rush from one activity to the next, many fall prone to neck, shoulder and back pain. The cobra posture minimises this pain by assisting to improve the flexibility of the nerves and reducing stress and stiffness in the ligaments. Through the practice of proper breathing mental equipoise will be developed and this will have a relaxing effect on these areas as well.

It benefits the whole nervous system, especially invigorating and strengthening the sciatic nerves and the nerves between the throat and brain.

The cobra increases the muscle tolerance of the arms and wrists and helps to remove problems with the ligaments and joints from an early age.

BENEFITS   COBRA POSTURE

Bhújaungásana activates the whole of the abdominal area from inside by giving pressure from the stomach outwardly.

Because of this gradual pressure and activation, the pancreas liver and other organs of the digestive system are strengthened and normalized.

It is regarded as one of the best asana for curing wind problem, indigestion, constipation, stomachache, dysentery and other abdominal disorders.

A variety of menstrual problem can be corrected by this ásana. If someone suffers from irregular menstruation or gets pains in the area of back and stomach for this reason, one should do this ásana twice in a day regularly.

Very few ásanas are prescribed for patients with high blood pressure. This ásana is one of the few which can be performed by them.

This ásana is also good for the liver.

This is one of the compulsory ásanas for women.

tuládandásana
BALANCE POSTURE

In Saṁskṛta tuládandá means scale as the body in this posture takes the appearance of a scale. This ásana is commonly known as balance posture in English.

Standing on the left foot, slowly raise the right foot backward. In order to keep balance place the hands on the waist and then bending the trunk and the head forward extend the leg until the body is parallel to the ground. Whilst gazing down the eyes should be fixed at a particular point. Keep the breathing regular and hold for thirty seconds

Standing on the right foot, repeat the process. One round consists of both legs. Practise four rounds.

6 BENEFITS

As the English name suggests the balance posture aids in finding a balance both in the physical and psychic levels and between the body and mind.

In today's society many people are suffering from emotional and psychic problems. These people may be single parents, struggling to bring up their children or part of the countless numbers who are unemployed and unable to progress in life. Quite often those who are under such pressures lose their clarity of thought as the mind becomes stuck in a spiral of despair. By practising this balancing posture the mind becomes more concentrated,

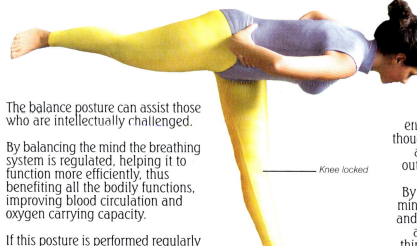

Knee locked

Feet placed firmly on the ground

The balance posture can assist those who are intellectually challenged.

By balancing the mind the breathing system is regulated, helping it to function more efficiently, thus benefiting all the bodily functions, improving blood circulation and oxygen carrying capacity.

If this posture is performed regularly it helps those suffering from sciatic pain, and by putting gentle pressure on the spine it relieves those with back pain.

enabling one to collect the thoughts of a scattered mind, and take a more positive outlook or approach to life.

By balancing the body, the mind becomes more focused and one-pointed, leading to an improvement in one's thinking capacity. This is of much benefit to those whose work entails mental exertion and especially helpful for those studying or employed in the academic field.

7

BENEFITS

The locust posture is of great benefit to women who suffer from menstrual pain.

It is good for relieving gout in the hands and feet and when performed regularly the locust alleviates rheumatism especially in the fingers and toes.

In Yoga science it is widely accepted that the root of many sicknesses lies in the stomach and intestine. Over eating or the consumption of the 'wrong' food can lead to undigested food sitting and eventually decomposing in the intestinal tract causing the build up of various toxins, poisoning the whole body and making one more prone to illness. The locust posture helps alleviate constipation, cures acidity and releases wind, thus acting as a deterrent to the formation of toxins and so is a preventative measure for further sickness.

If one becomes accustomed to practising this posture one will fortify the veins and nerves of the upper legs, making them extremely strong and thus able to walk over long distances.

shalabhásana

In Saṁskṛta shalabha means locust.

Lie face down keeping the arms to the side of the body. Take long and steady breaths relaxing the entire body.

STEP 1

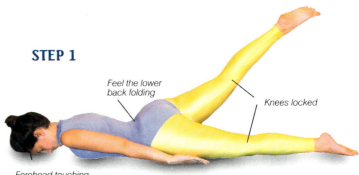

Feel the lower back folding
Knees locked
Forehead touching the ground

Inhale and at the same time lift the right leg using the support of the hands on the ground. One may also clench the hands into fists for extra leverage. Hold this position for thirty seconds breathing freely yet steadily, and then lower the leg to the ground.

STEP 2

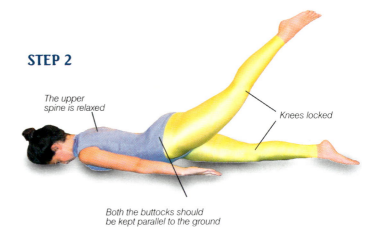

The upper spine is relaxed
Knees locked
Both the buttocks should be kept parallel to the ground

Repeat step 1, this time lifting the left leg.

LOCUST POSTURE

When practised frequently and properly the locust posture helps to reduce weight around the thighs and buttocks, and is particularly beneficial for removing cellulite, as it exercises the muscles and aids the blood circulation in the legs.

STEP 3

From lying position inhale slowly and without bending the knees lift both the legs as high as possible.

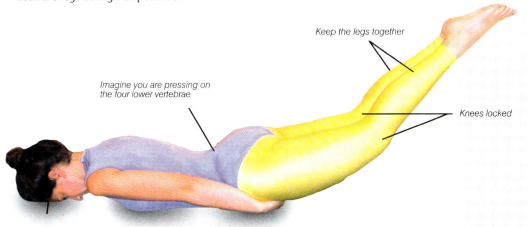

Keep the legs together

Imagine you are pressing on the four lower vertebrae

Knees locked

Forehead on the ground

Feel the stretch on the lower four vertebrae of the spine. Hold this position for thirty seconds with regular breathing then slowly return the legs to the ground.

In the beginning you may not be able to lift the legs properly but with regular practice you can progress quickly and derive many benefits from this posture.

It bolsters the upper portion of the body above the navel, invigorating the heart and lungs, and benefits the upper part of the spine, exercising the first four vertebrae of the spinal column that the cobra posture does not reach.

CAUTION:
Those who suffer from heart and lungs problem or hypertension should not perform this ásana. Pregnant women should also avoid this posture.

8 nāokāsana

Naoká means boat in Saṁskṛta and this ásana is referred to as the boat or bow posture in English.

BENEFITS

By practising the boat posture one applies pressure on the stomach, which serves to reduce any excess fat in that area and activates both the large and small intestine, the spleen and the liver.

This ásana helps rid the body of indigestion and gout and relieves those suffering from dyspepsia, rheumatism and other gastro- intestinal disorders. Generally these disorders are brought on by the accumulation of toxins in the body. By performing the boat posture one helps to eliminate these poisons.

By practising the boat regularly one's appetite will increase, and laziness in the body and mind will be overcome.

This posture massages all the nerve fibres and muscles in the back, while specifically fortifying the middle portion of the spine.

When one follows the proper breathing system prescribed with this ásana it has a tremendous benefit on the lungs, helping to alleviate asthmatic disorders.

The effect of the boat posture on the manipura cakra assists in balancing the secretion of hormones from the adrenal glands, removing stress, fear and tension and instilling peace to an otherwise restless mind.

It strengthens the muscles of the legs and arms creating balance between the middle portion of the body and the lower portion.

By performing this posture one massages the entire body and benefits all aspects of the physical structure.

If someone is regular in doing Cobra, Locust and Boat posture, one should start from cobra and finish with the wheel posture. Though it is not a hard and fast rule, it is better to follow this sequence.

BOAT POSTURE

STEP 1

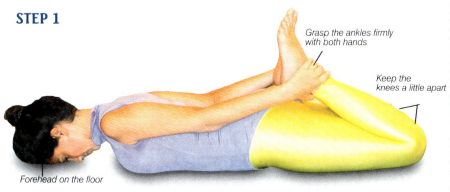

Grasp the ankles firmly with both hands

Keep the knees a little apart

Forehead on the floor

STEP 2

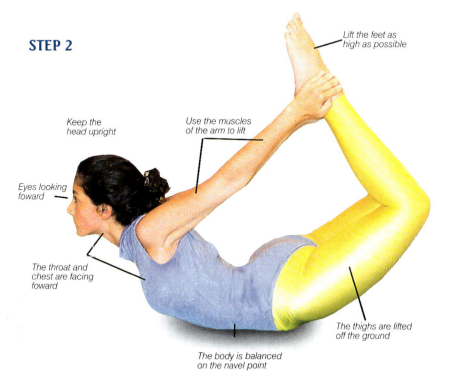

Lift the feet as high as possible

Keep the head upright

Use the muscles of the arm to lift

Eyes looking foward

The throat and chest are facing foward

The thighs are lifted off the ground

The body is balanced on the navel point

METHOD

Lie face down and regulate your breathing. Bring the lower legs close to the thighs and directing the hands over the back grasp the ankles. Inhale while raising the entire body, supporting the weight on the navel. Extend the neck and chest as far back as possible. Keep the eyes directed forward.

Maintain this position for eight seconds and then while exhaling resume the original posture. In this manner practise this ásana eight times. In this ásana the body should assume the shape of a bow.

Please note that yoga ásanas are not meant to be parctised to the point of exhaustion. If one practises these postures slowly and gradually in a systematic way they will have a tremendous relaxing effect on both the body and mind.

67

9

cakrāsana

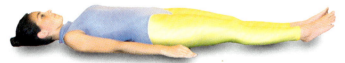

In Saṁskṛta cakra means wheel. This āsana is commonly known as the wheel or bridge posture.

BENEFITS

This āsana has an invigorating effect on the whole of digestive system. By regularly practising this āsana one may alleviate problems with constipation and indigestion.

It cures calcification in the back, removing rheumatic problems and lower back pain.

This posture helps to cure men's disorders such as impotency and loss of semen.

It has a strengthening effect on the lungs, helping to improve one's stamina

With frequent performance this posture brings a shining glow, helping to reduce fat as it massages the whole spinal column.

If practised from childhood, or before the age of fifteen, it helps to prevent stunted growth and dwarfism.

STEP 1

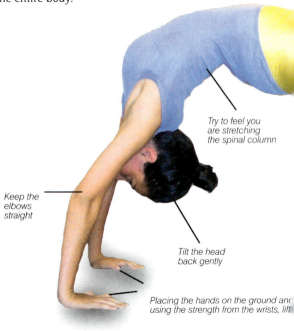

Lie on your back with the arms to the side and breathing deeply relax the entire body.

Try to feel you are stretching the spinal column

Keep the elbows straight

Tilt the head back gently

Placing the hands on the ground and using the strength from the wrists, lift

STEP 2

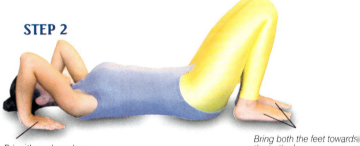

Bring the palms close to the ears

Bring both the feet towards the buttocks

Flex the legs, bringing the lower legs in close contact to the thighs. Place both the hands close to the ears, palms down.

WHEEL POSTURE

STEP 3
Supporting the weight on the soles and the palms, gradually raise the entire body off the ground. Pay attention to the hands and feet as you utilize their strength to gradually lift the body as high as possible.

This ásana stretches the spine allowing the energy to flow freely to the brain. Due to this nourishment the brain's functions are improved resulting in a higher level of intelligence. This posture should be encouraged in children.

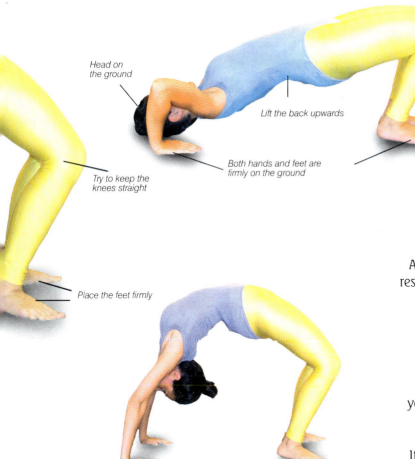

Head on the ground

Lift the back upwards

Both hands and feet are firmly on the ground

Try to keep the knees straight

Place the feet firmly

After child-birth, it helps to reshape any looseness in the mother's stomach.

It works to strengthen the palms, wrists and elbows.

It helps one to maintain youthfulness by halting the aging process.

It is a good ásana for those suffering from diabetes.

STEP 4
The body will assume the shape of a wheel in this ásana, with the hands and feet kept parallel to each other. Let the breath flow freely and hold this position for thirty seconds. Practise four times.

WARNING! This ásana should never be practised during pregnancy.

10

BENEFITS

This ásana works with the lower three cakras.

It removes gas from the stomach and helps alleviate constipation and headaches.

The bellows posture has the power to cure many types of intestinal problems

It has greater benefit when practised in the morning. Before starting your day do this posture and then take one glass of water or grapefruit juice. By combining this exercise and drinking system one will be able to clear the bowels thoroughly, leaving the body and mind clear and light.

> Follow the same gesture with the same breathing technique with the right leg.

bhastrikásana
BELLOWS POSTURE

Bhastriká means bellows. This posture is highly recommended for the stomach and intestines.

STEP 1

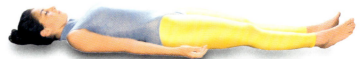

Lie on your back in a relaxed state.

STEP 2

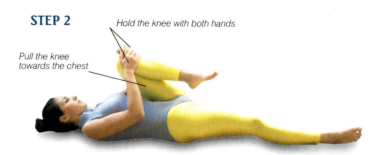

Hold the knee with both hands

Pull the knee towards the chest

While breathing out, bend the left leg and bring the thigh into contact with the chest. Grasp the leg firmly with both hands. Maintain this position for eight seconds, holding the out breath.

STEP 3

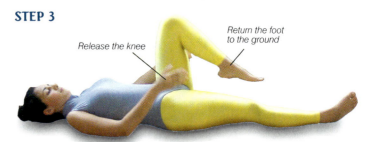

Release the knee

Return the foot to the ground

Breathing in, release the left leg, resuming the original position. Practise similarly with the right leg, and then both legs together.

STEP 4

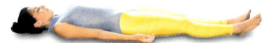

One complete round is comprised of three parts; the right leg, the left leg, and both legs together.

Practise eight such rounds, that is
8 x 3 = 24 positions

utkśepa mudrá
UTKŚEPA MUDRÁ

11

Lie flat on the back in a relaxed position.

STEP 1

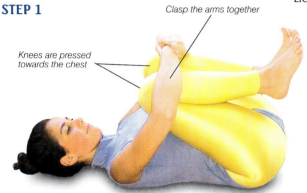

Clasp the arms together

Knees are pressed towards the chest

Bring both the knees to the chest. Grasp the knees with the arms and steadily press them tight to the chest. At the same time inhale and maintain this posture for eight seconds.

STEP 2

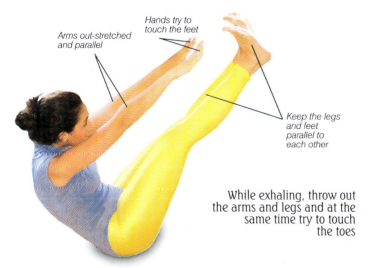

Arms out-stretched and parallel

Hands try to touch the feet

Keep the legs and feet parallel to each other

While exhaling, throw out the arms and legs and at the same time try to touch the toes

This posture should be performed first thing in the morning, before rising from bed. Then taking one glass of water or juice, expose the navel area to the air and walk for a while. This combination will have the effect of cleaning the bowels.

While performing this mudrá one will automatically attain the benefit of Bhastrikásana.

To accelerate the cleaning of the bowels one should concentrate on the stomach area when practising this posture, try to feel that all the organs such as the pancreas, stomach and bowels are operating correctly.

When performing this posture one should keep silent and concentrate the mind. This will have a calming effect on both the body and mind helping one to get maximum benefit from this ásana.

Before beginning this posture one should take a number of long and deep breaths and then thrust out the legs

Utkśepa mudrá has the capacity to cure many stomach problems, and also removes hard constipation.

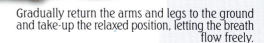

Gradually return the arms and legs to the ground and take-up the relaxed position, letting the breath flow freely.

Practise three or four times.

12 shasháungásana

BENEFITS

This posture is of great benefit to the veins and nerves of the back, making one's spine very supple.

It maintains the heat of the pancreas and is very beneficial for the tonsils.

It fortifies all the cakras and the glands of the entire body, helping to balance the secretion of hormones throughout.

If one practices this ásana from childhood, one can increase the height of the body.

As the backbone gets stretched, it becomes very flexible.

It nourishes the nervous system of the body.

It increases the beauty and luster of the body and it prolongs a youthful life.

It has the capacity to improve the digestion system.

It helps to get appetite, removes insomnia.

In Saṁskṛta, Shasha means hare.

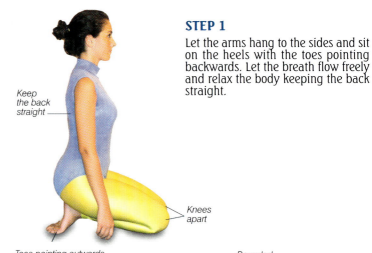

Keep the back straight
Toes pointing outwards
Knees apart
Rounded back
Grasp the heels
Head touches the knees

STEP 1
Let the arms hang to the sides and sit on the heels with the toes pointing backwards. Let the breath flow freely and relax the body keeping the back straight.

STEP 2
Grasp the heels and exhaling, bring the crown of the head to the floor placing the head between the knees.

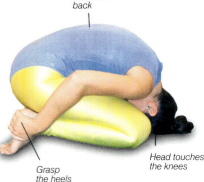

Keep the hips up
Head touches the floor between the knees
The body will take an elliptical shape

STEP 3
Continue exhaling and at the same time lift the buttocks pressing the head gently on the ground.

HARE POSTURE

It influences both the thyroid and parathyroid glands and it removes the bad breath.

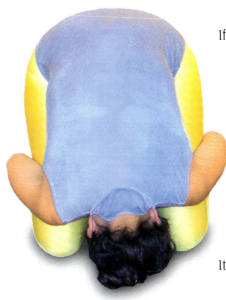

If there is a burning sensation in the ear, this ásana can relieve it.

Maintain this position for eight seconds. Inhale as you raise the head and return to the kneeling position. Repeat six to eight times.

It is good for developing pleasing and sound voice.

It helps to cure epilepsy, reduce body fat and is specifically good for the development of the thyroid gland.

It has the capacity to improve one's memory, making the mind introverted and helps with concentration and meditation.

This ásana is considered the fourth best after the shoulder stand, the twist and full-head-to-knee postures.

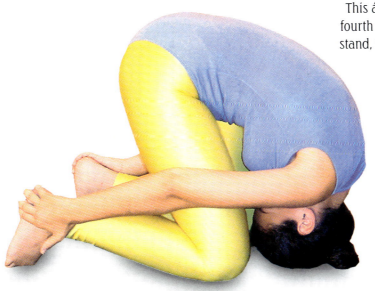

CAUTION
Those who have cervical spondylosis should not do this posture.

Please note that those who have high blood pressure, or who are pregnant should avoid this ásana.

13

uṣṭrāsana

Uṣṭra means camel in saṁskṛta. As the chest is lifted in this posture it takes the form of a camel's hump. Like the camel that possesses the strength and stamina to endure heavy loads, this posture will endow the practitioner with added strength and stamina.

STEP 1

Kneel down with the toes pointing backwards and let the breath flow freely for a short time.

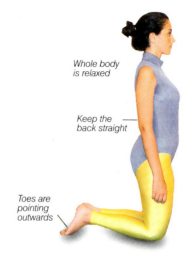

Whole body is relaxed

Keep the back straight

Toes are pointing outwards

STEP 2

Inhaling gently bend the body backwards. At the same time rotate each arm over the head and touch the heels. Tilting the head backwards extend the chest and stomach.

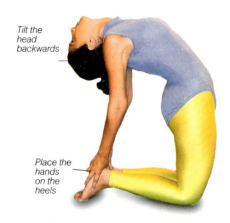

Tilt the head backwards

Place the hands on the heels

BENEFITS

This exercise has a positive effect on the vertebrae, strengthening the nerves and nerve fibres of this area.

With regular practice this posture helps the body remain youthful and if started at an early age, it can increase one's height.

When performing this āsana one should concentrate on breathing deeply and this will have a strengthening effect on the respiratory system.

This āsana is cleansing for the lungs clearing out unwanted phlegm and bile.

Those who suffer from diabetes should practise this āsana. It is greatly beneficial for those with lower back pain.

It has a rejuvenating effect on the neck, shoulders and spine, and with regular practice, it can make one's chest shapely.

CAMEL POSTURE

STEP 3

Lift the torso until it takes the shape of the camel's hump. As you raise your body inhale deeply and try to touch the fingers to the toes. After touching the toes you may feel the energy circulating around the body. This posture naturally helps to create a flow of bio-energy in the body.

The practice of touching the toes with the fingers will help the circulation of energy in the body. One will feel that the bio-energy system of the body is enriched.

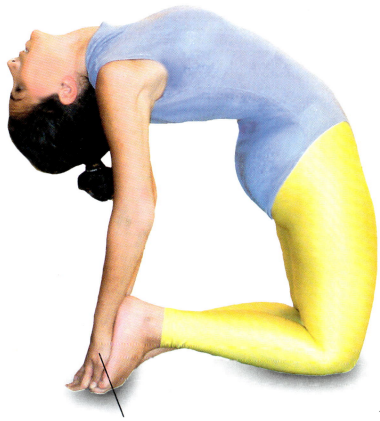

The palms touch the soles of the feet

This ásana improves the eyesight, cures headache, is good for the tonsils, and helps to maintain celibacy.

Hold your breath in this ásana eight seconds, then exhaling return to the kneeling position.
Repeat this posture four to six times.

The camel posture alleviates cacophony or harshness of the voice.

14

BENEFITS

Regular practice of this ásana makes one as strong as thunder, especially stretching and strengthening the area around the waist.

It is most beneficial for those suffering from sciatica and gout.

It revitalizes the sex organs and when performed regularly one will be able to keep the colour of the hair.

It strengthens the spine helping to maintain youthfulness, and promoting longevity.

Keeping the breath regular, practice this posture cautiously and with perseverance the body's ligaments will soon loosen.
Clench the fists and place them upon the knees.

Keep the arms straight with the head and back erect.
Practise four rounds, thirty seconds each time.

Vajrásana
THUNDER POSTURE

In Saṁskṛta Vajra means thunder.

Sit on the floor with the ankles to the side, feet pointing outwards. In the beginning if you find difficulty sitting in this posture you may like to practise on a softer surface (such as pillows).

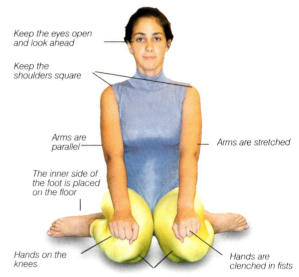

Keep the eyes open and look ahead
Keep the shoulders square
Arms are parallel
Arms are stretched
The inner side of the foot is placed on the floor
Hands on the knees
Hands are clenched in fists
Arms are extended forward

Starting pose for utkaṭa vajrásana

Sit in Vajrásana and taking the support of the forearms gradually lower the body with the head tilting backwards. Lie down fully taking the support of the palms.

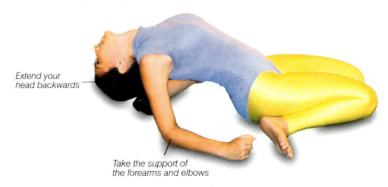

Extend your head backwards
Take the support of the forearms and elbows

utkata vajrāsana
DIFFICULT THUNDER POSTURE

15
BENEFITS

STEP 1
Place the hands behind the head with the fingers interlocked.

Difficult thunder posture possesses all the benefits of Vajrāsana.

It strengthens and develops the nervous system of the body making the veins flexible yet tough.

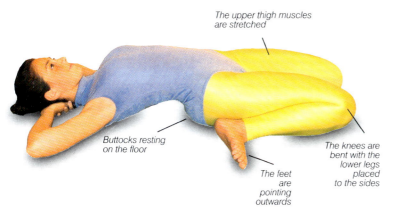

The upper thigh muscles are stretched

Buttocks resting on the floor

The knees are bent with the lower legs placed to the sides

The feet are pointing outwards

This āsana counters all sorts of back pain helping to keep the elasticity of the spine. It is considered the best posture for healing diabetes.

It is good for the pancreas, improving its function

STEP 2
Stretch the arms backwards, touching the ears and try to feel the deep stretch along the whole spine.

The regular practice of this posture will balance the acid reaction in the stomach thus invigorating the whole of the body's digestion system.

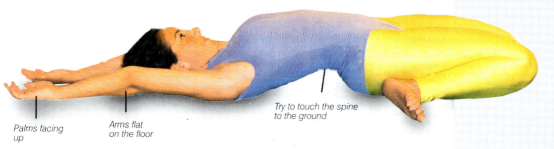

Palms facing up

Arms flat on the floor

Try to touch the spine to the ground

This āsana can also be practiced for its relaxation benefits.

77

16 gomukhāsana

In Saṁskṛta `go` means cow and `mukha` is head, so this is the cow's head posture

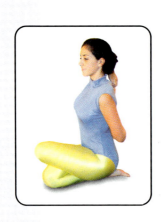

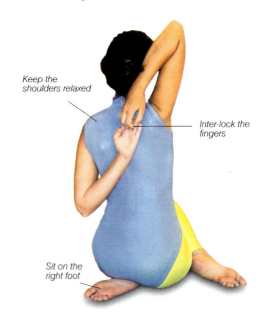

- Keep the shoulders relaxed
- Inter-lock the fingers
- Sit on the right foot

Sit down and extend the legs forward.

Bring the right leg under the left thigh.

Place the right foot under the left buttock.

Put the left leg across the right thigh.

Keep the back erect.

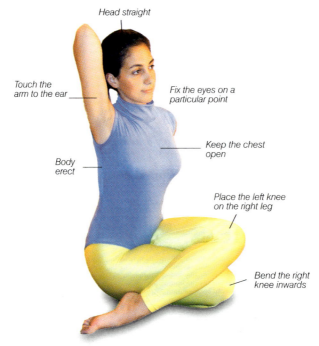

- Head straight
- Touch the arm to the ear
- Fix the eyes on a particular point
- Keep the chest open
- Body erect
- Place the left knee on the right leg
- Bend the right knee inwards

Bring the left hand behind and place it on the spine.

Then bring the right hand backward over the right shoulder.

Inter-lock the fingers of the hands.

Hold for thirty seconds with regular breathing.

One round consists of both left and right sides

COW'S HEAD POSTURE

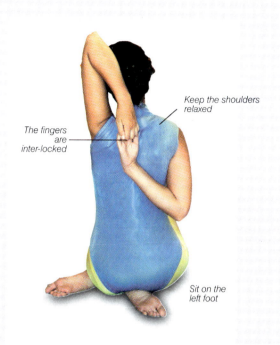

The fingers are inter-locked

Keep the shoulders relaxed

Sit on the left foot

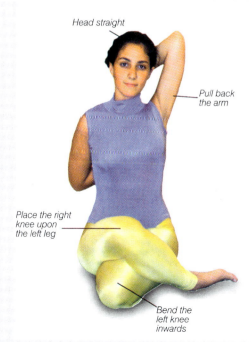

Head straight

Pull back the arm

Place the right knee upon the left leg

Bend the left knee inwards

Try to keep the back erect and the head straight.

Keep the eyes focussed on a point in front.

Practise the same way with the left leg under the right.

While performing this ásana try to keep the breathing steady, relaxing the whole body.

Perform four rounds

BENEFITS

The cow's head stretches and strengthens the shoulder muscles, massaging the vertebrae, and thus helping to ease back problems.

It provides great relief to those suffering from rheumatism and arthritis, and can be of help in curing tumours.

This posture relieves gout, sciatica, piles, and any burning sensation inside the urinary duct.

Regular practice helps to develop the chest, lungs and heart as well as benefiting the kidneys and is considered one of the best ásanas for curing insomnia.

Gomukhásana aids those with sexual problems having the power to remove impure thoughts.

This ásana is particularly beneficial in removing constipation and dyspepsia, helping to create a healthy appetite.

It is especially good for sickly persons that often suffer from fevers and colds.

Please note: women should try to avoid this ásana and if they do practise it, they should proceed with caution.

17 baddha padmāsana

In Saṁskṛta 'baddha' means to bind, and padma is lotus. So this is the bound lotus posture.

BENEFITS

This āsana has all the benefits of lotus posture helping to straighten and strengthen the spine so that one can sit straight.

By following a deep breathing system one will strengthen and increase the capacity of the lungs.

This āsana is the best tonic for lethargy and idleness taking away feelings of sleepiness and having the power to make the mind active and introverted. This posture strengthens the muscles of the hands and arms helping to reduce weight around the waist.

This posture strengthens the muscles of the neck and shoulders and helps to remove the calcification in those areas.

Those whose shoulders are not parallel to each other, they should practice this posture regularly.

It removes the pain in knee and heels.

It also has the benefit of removing weakness in the legs.

STEP 1
Sit in Lotus posture.

Head straight
Keep the body erect
Place the feet on top of the legs

STEP 2
Direct the left hand backwards from the left side and grasp the big toe of the left foot.

The left hand grasps the big toe

BOUND LOTUS POSTURE

With regular practice, this ásana will make one bold and self-confident.

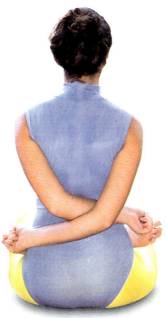

STEP 3
Then direct the right hand behind and grasp the big toe of the right foot. Gently pull on the toes at the same time straightening the head, shoulders and back. Thrust the chest forward.

While doing this posture take deep breaths and try to imagine that the cells in your brain are being nourished. Inhaling imagine you are expanding your entire mind.
Maintain this posture for thirty seconds. Practise four times.

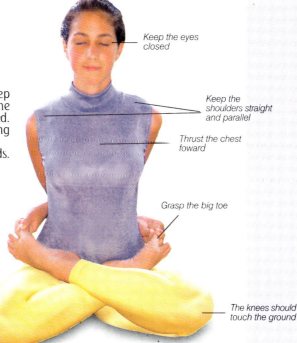

Keep the eyes closed

Keep the shoulders straight and parallel

Thrust the chest foward

Grasp the big toe

The knees should touch the ground

18 jánushirásana

In Saṁskṛta 'jánu' means knee and 'shira' means head. So this is named the head to knee posture.

BENEFITS

Halfhead-to-knee ásana increases one's digestion capacity, strengthening the maṅipura cakra.

This posture is particularly beneficial for those suffering from colic pain, sciatica and piles. It vitalises the nerves and veins of the navel area and helps to remove idleness.

It also strengthens and stretches the lower back helping to alleviate lower back pain.

This ásana massages the thymus gland helping to balance the secretion of hormones.

If one cannot reach the toes grasp the ankles and gradually try to touch the head to the knee.

One should avoid this posture if one has a headache.

It is the best cure for the early stage of lumbago pain.

It also removes laziness, slough and is an antidote for a sedentary life-style.

STEP 1
Sit with the back erect and legs outstretched. Fold the right leg and place the right foot against the left thigh. Take slow deep breaths

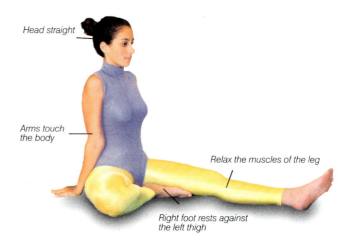

Head straight
Arms touch the body
Relax the muscles of the leg
Right foot rests against the left thigh

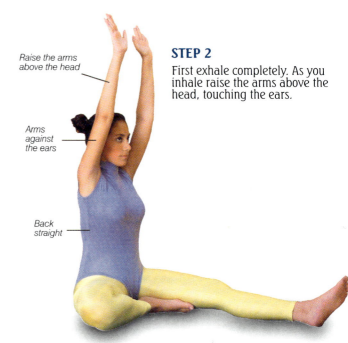

Raise the arms above the head
Arms against the ears
Back straight

STEP 2
First exhale completely. As you inhale raise the arms above the head, touching the ears.

HEAD TO KNEE POSTURE

STEP 3
Very calmly and steadily exhale bringing down the arms, taking hold of the toes and resting the head upon the knee. Try to keep the left leg straight. Maintain this position for eight seconds while holding the out breath.

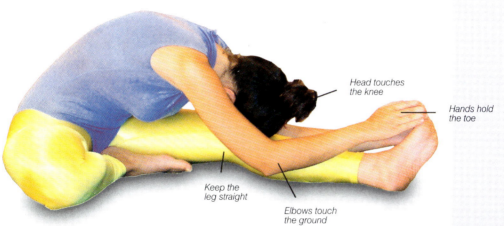

Head touches the knee

Hands hold the toe

Keep the leg straight

Elbows touch the ground

It makes the lower portion of the spinal cord very flexible.

It helps to increase the body's length for those who are born as dwarf. Provided it is practiced from 12 years old.

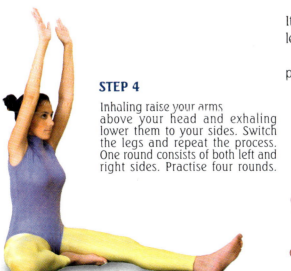

STEP 4
Inhaling raise your arms above your head and exhaling lower them to your sides. Switch the legs and repeat the process. One round consists of both left and right sides. Practise four rounds.

CAUTION:
Those who have high blood pressure or cardiovascular diseases should avoid doing this ásana.

19 pashcimottánásana

BENEFITS

Pashcimottánásana makes the lower portion of the body strong and increases the flexibility of the knees.

This ásana is beneficial for stretching the spine to its maximum capacity, removing painful compressions in the nerves. With regular practice, this ásana beautifies and tones the body, removing excess fat.

It has the power to remove acidity in the blood.

This ásana works on the spleen, appendix and kidney and is especially helpful for the sciatic nerve.

The fullhead-to-knee helps one with urinary problems, specifically the inability to control the bladder. On the psycho-physical level this ásana helps to increase one's tolerance to pain, especially strengthening the first and second cakras.

Here Saṁskṛta pashcima means the lower portion of the body. The posture, by which lower portion of the body is strengthened, that is called pashcimottánásana. In English this posture is commonly known as full head to knee.

STEP 1
Lie down on your back. Bring the arms backwards touching the ears. Relax keeping the breath flowing freely.

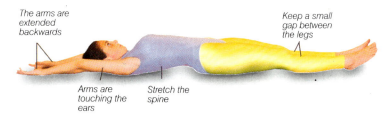

The arms are extended backwards
Arms are touching the ears
Stretch the spine
Keep a small gap between the legs

STEP 2
Inhale and then exhale raising the body, keeping the arms straight and touching the ears.

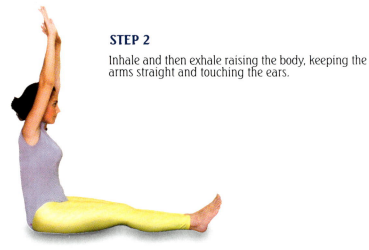

STEP 3
Continue to exhale, lower the body, grasping the toes and placing the head between the knees.

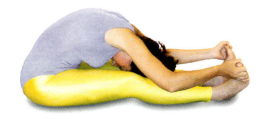

FULLHEAD TO KNEE

Place the head between the legs with the elbows touching the ground. Try to keep the knees straight. Hold for eight seconds also holding the out breath.

It is one of the ásanas prescribed for those suffering from diabetes.

It helps to remove dreams of a sexual nature.

This ásana is considered the third best after the shoulder stand and twist postures.

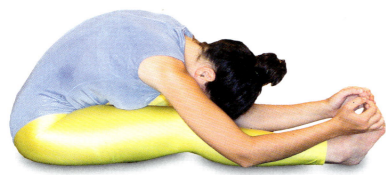

After eight seconds inhale and keeping the arms outstretched raise your body and return to a lying position. This posture should be practised eight times.

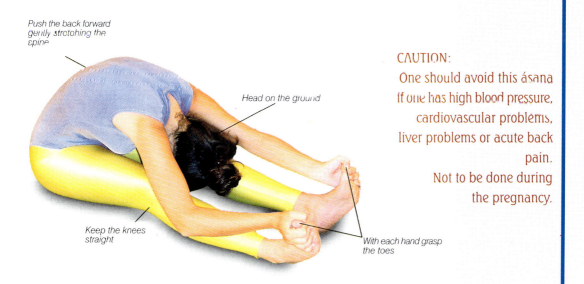

Push the back forward gently stretching the spine

Head on the ground

Keep the knees straight

With each hand grasp the toes

CAUTION:
One should avoid this ásana if one has high blood pressure, cardiovascular problems, liver problems or acute back pain.
Not to be done during the pregnancy.

20 Ekapadashiirṣāsana

BENEFITS

This is one of the best āsanas to keep the body ever flexible, helping to maintain a strong back, developing the muscles and nerves of the legs and generally benefiting the hands, arms, feet and neck.

It is especially good for the kidneys and the adrenal glands helping to regulate the metabolism and control any hyper-active tendencies.

It strengthens the third cakra by applying pressure on the navel point thus energising the whole body.

With regular practice this āsana will help balance the hormone secretion and maintain a healthy balance between body and mind.

The benefits to this pose are so extensive that if one can manage to place both legs behind the head at once there is no need to practise any other āsana.

Sit comfortably on the floor and concentrate on your breathing.

Like Granthimuktāsana this āsana rids the body of toxins, especially in the leg joints. One can attain tremendous benefits by placing the foot behind the neck.
This posture should be performed gradually, first bringing the leg towards the stomach, then lifting towards the ear and then finally placing behind the neck.
When the heel of the foot comes behind the head one may bend the head forward a little to accommodate.

STEP 1

Sit straight with both the legs extended in front. With both the hands grasp the left foot and pull towards you. Gradually lift the foot and place it behind the neck. With the right hand grasp the toes of the left foot. Try to sit straight and look ahead.

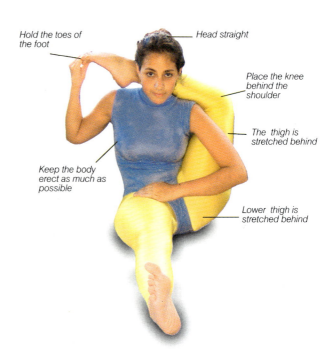

Hold the toes of the foot
Head straight
Place the knee behind the shoulder
The thigh is stretched behind
Keep the body erect as much as possible
Lower thigh is stretched behind

FOOT TO HEAD POSTURE

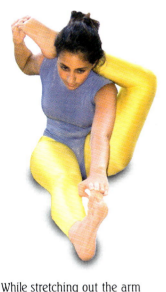

STEP 2

While placing the foot behind the neck and grasping the toes with the right hand, let the left arm come forward and grab the toes. The knee of the outstretched leg should be kept straight.

This ásana increases the digestion capacity.

With regular practice, one can be free from wind problem in the stomach. Also it is good for liver and spleen.

If one continuously practises this pose, one will not get wrinkles even in later life after age fifty.

It removes lethargic tendency.

While stretching out the arm to touch the toes of the outstretched leg one should exhale. Hold for eight seconds then release. Use both hands and carefully lower the foot and leg from behind the neck. One round is equal to both legs. Repeat four to six times.

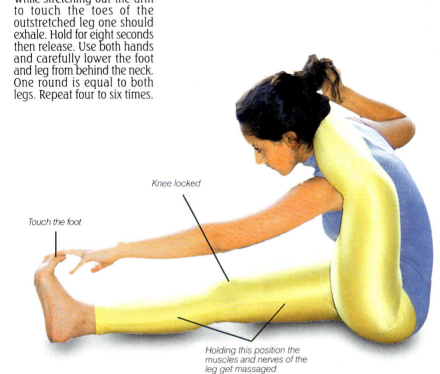

Touch the foot

Knee locked

Holding this position the muscles and nerves of the leg get massaged

Matsyendrāsana

21

BENEFITS

This posture massages the veins, arteries and nerves of the back, leading to increased flexibility

It is a good posture for lower back pain, curing any arthritis in the back and allowing the spine to rejuvenate.

The twist removes constipation and dyspepsia.

This posture influences all the sensory and motor organs, activates all the cakras and brings mental peace and calmness.

It is good for those suffering from diabetes

With regular practice it helps to prevent the calcification of the vertebrae, maintaining the body's youthfulness, and increasing longevity

This āsana was invented by a great ṛṣi by the name of Matsyendranāth, who had achieved the occult power to attract the rain. It is more commonly called the `spinal twist`

STEP 1
Bend the knee of the right leg and sit on the right foot.

Balance the body

Sit on the right foot

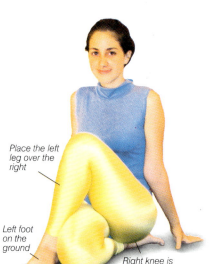

Place the left leg over the right

Left foot on the ground

Right knee is bent

STEP 2
Cross the left foot over the right thigh, keeping the body straight.

STEP 3
Grasp the left toe with the right arm keeping the right arm along the left side of the left knee. To effectively perform this āsana one must gradually twist the waist into the correct position.

The upper portion of the arm presses against the knee

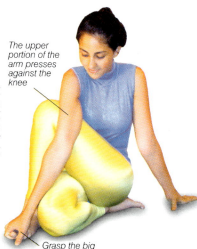

Grasp the big toe

SPINAL TWIST

STEP 4

Reach behind with the left hand and touch the navel area. At the same time turn the head to the left turning the eyes toward the elbow of the left arm. The breath should be free flowing and natural.

Reverse the process pressing the múládhára cakra with the left heel. One round means completing the process on both sides. Practise four rounds.

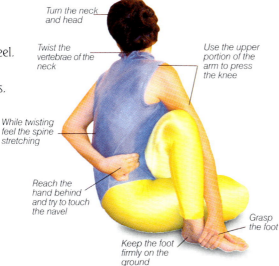

Turn the neck and head
Twist the vertebrae of the neck
Use the upper portion of the arm to press the knee
While twisting feel the spine stretching
Reach the hand behind and try to touch the navel
Grasp the foot
Keep the foot firmly on the ground

The spinal twist is one of the fundamental ásanas for men and after the shoulder-stand the twist is considered the most beneficial ásana, helping one to perform pashcimottánásana.

If one is short of time then practising this ásana gives an all-round benefit, which can be felt for a long period after finishing your routine.

It helps the blood circulate around the body, re-energising the cells and tissues.

By looking at the elbow in this posture one can attain peace of mind.

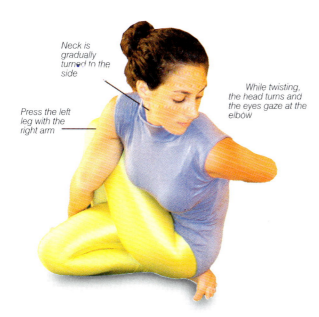

Neck is gradually turned to the side
Press the left leg with the right arm
While twisting, the head turns and the eyes gaze at the elbow

CAUTION:
Women should avoid practising this posture during pregnancy and menstruation.

22 sarváungásana

BENEFITS

This ásana is a panacea for all diseases, at the same time developing and resting all the glands of the body.

It is one of the most valued ásana of the hatha yoga system.

As its name indicates it is indeed a posture of the whole body.

There is hardly any portion of the body which is not energized, exercised, or activated. For this reason it is one of the best of all the ásanas.

By activating all the glands of the body this ásana acts as a preventative measure for many sicknesses.

This posture is of particular benefit to the thyroid and parathyroid glands, helping also to alleviate tonsillitis.

It helps in cholera, small-pox, typhoid and pneumonia cases as well as those who are suffering from leprosy.

The candle-stick posture relieves constipation and spleen related problems.

In Samskrta 'sarva' means all and áunga means limbs, therefore this is the all limbs posture. Because one stands with the strength of the shoulders this position is commonly known as the shoulder-stand.

From a relaxed position lift the legs and hold at a thirty-degree angle. Then repeat the process this time lifting the legs to a ninety-degree angle.
To complete the shoulder-stand raise the entire body straight into the air with the legs straight. Rest the entire weight on the body's shoulders supporting both the sides of the trunk with the hands. The higher up the torso one can hold the hands the straighter the posture. The chin should touch the chest and keeping the feet together, direct the gaze at the toes.

This posture should be alternated with Matsyamudrá or fish gesture. Practising the shoulder-stand with the fish posture is considered one round. Though many practitioners only do shoulder-stand it is not recommended, as the thyroid gland is activated in shoulder-stand and to balance the parathyroid gland should be activated in the fish. The fish posture should be practised for half the duration of the shoulder-stand. For example, if one does one minute of shoulder stand the fish should be practised for thirty seconds. Practise three rounds.

STEP 1

Lie down on your back.
Relax all the limbs of your body.
Wait a bit, till your breath is fully normalized and your mind
completely balanced and concentrated.

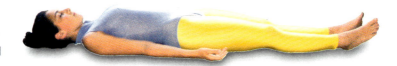

If one is unable to complete the full all limbs posture with the chin touching the chest then lifting the body as high as possible still has great benefit.
If the all limbs posture is practised properly all the cakras and glands are activated especially the thyroid and parathyroid. The moment the body is inverted the glands are able to take rest and the blood circulation is intensified helping to balance the hormone secretion in the entire body.

ALL LIMBS POSTURE

STEP 2

Raise the legs firmly and hands. The chin angle of the body Maintain this position with up at the toes. The weight of on the shoulders.

In your yoga routine, if you are it is better to perform

supporting the body with the arms should touch the chest. The should be ninety degrees. regular breathing, looking the whole body should rest

doing, more than 3-4 ásanas, Sarvauṅgásana at the end.

It alleviates many diseases specific to women including displaced uterus.

It removes physical debility, headache and piles, as well as alleviating shooting pains in the body.

It increases the longevity of a person and is extremely beneficial for obesity

It benefits those who suffer from anaemia

It helps those who suffer from excess sleeping.

The Sarváuṅgásana is a complete ásana, which helps one to activate all the limbs, as it is called 'Sarváuṅgásana'.

One must warm up the body, get the muscles elastic, and then start doing more difficult postures like Sarváuṅgásana. Otherwise, one may become a victim of cramps.

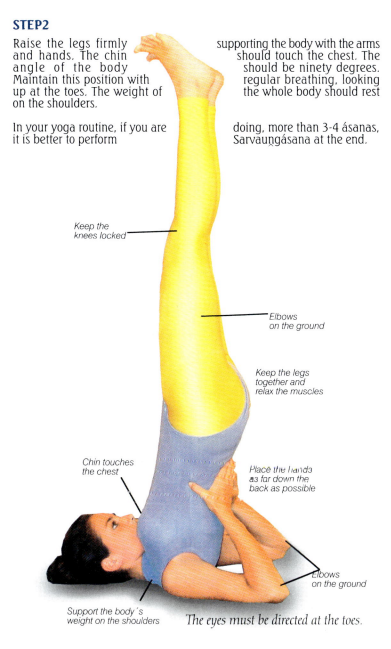

- Keep the knees locked
- Elbows on the ground
- Keep the legs together and relax the muscles
- Chin touches the chest
- Place the hands as far down the back as possible
- Elbows on the ground
- Support the body's weight on the shoulders

The eyes must be directed at the toes.

CAUTION:
This posture should not be done by those over the age of sixty or who have high blood pressure or heart problems.

While performing ásanas, we should remember to do the easier less complicated ásanas first, before the full and complete ásanas.

23

matsyamudrá

In Saṁskṛta matsya means fish and mudrá gesture, thus this is called the fish gesture.

BENEFITS

This ásana greatly benefits the respiratory system

It decompresses the thyroid and parathyroid glands balancing their hormone secretion

Beneficial for menstruation problems

It helps to release gas in the body relieving constipation

This posture has a positive effect on the pancreas.

This posture helps to retain calcium in the body. If there is low hormone secretion from the parathyroid gland then calcium is not absorbed and it will not be able to properly nourish the body. This leads to constipation, indigestion, gastric ulcer and pyorrhoea.

During the practice of this ásana, one places pressure upon the back.

The chest gets enlarged.

As a result of that, one can breathe in a better way

The posture strengthens the lungs.

STEP 1

Begin by sitting in lotus posture. If one is unable to perform lotus one may sit in a comfortable cross-legged position.

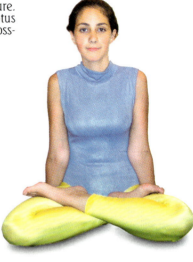

STEP 2

Taking the support of the forearms lean the body backwards and tilt the head back.

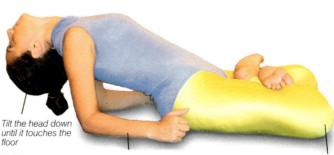

Tilt the head down until it touches the floor

Keep the forearm on the floor

Knees on the floor

FISH GESTURE

STEP 3

Lean back until the top of the head touches the ground, keeping the neck in full stretch. The back is arched with the chest thrust forward. Keeping the elbows on the floor clasp the toes with the hands. If one is a little overweight one can place a pillow under the back for support. The duration of this ásana depends on the amount of time spent in shoulder stand. If shoulder stand was maintained for three minutes then the fish gesture should be performed for one and a half minutes. Repeat three times.

It is good for asthma, cough and cold, bronchitis, tonsils etc.

If the structure of the chest is defective, one should do this ásana regularly beginning at an early age.

If someone has pain in the neck and waist, s/he should do it regularly.

It is helpful for headaches, mental fatigue and to some extend insomnia.

It helps in skin diseases, appendicitis, hernia, boils and acne.

This ásana activates the vishuddha cakra, benefiting the vocal cord.

It is very good for those afflicted with asthma.

The proper function of the Parathyroid and thyroid helps to maintain the whole body

It strengthens the teeth and gums by giving proper circulation in those places.

STEP 4

For those who have a problem sitting with the legs folded then one may keep the legs outstretched.

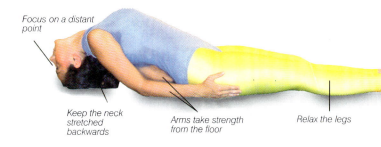

CAUTION:
Those who suffer from high blood pressure should avoid practising this ásana

24 halāsana

BENEFITS

As while doing this āsana, one has to pass through Sarvāungāsana. One gets almost all the benefits of Sarvāungāsana.

It strengthens the abdominal muscles and exercises all the vertebrae of the spine, stretching the whole spine and relieving lower back pain.

Halāsana can alleviate various types of neck pain, releasing any tension that may have accumulated in those areas.

It is good for the liver and spleen and gives relief to those suffering from muscular rheumatism.

Halāsana tones up the entire body especially helping those with obesity.

It is good for removing constipation and indigestion.

The plough develops patience, memory and higher consciousness.

In Saṁskṛta 'hala' means plough.

STEP 1

Lie down on the back and relax the entire body.

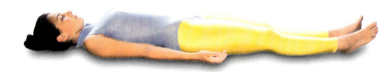

STEP 2

Rise to the position of the all limbs posture with the legs extended in the air and the chin touching the chest.

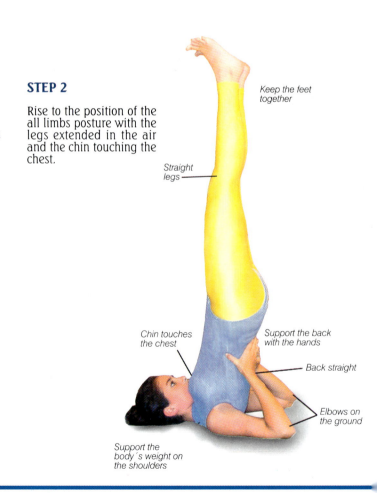

Keep the feet together

Straight legs

Chin touches the chest

Support the back with the hands

Back straight

Elbows on the ground

Support the body´s weight on the shoulders

THE PLOUGH

STEP 3

Gradually bring the legs backwards and extend them as far as possible. Let the toes touch the ground, keeping the arms in a prone position on either side of the body. Maintain this posture trying to feel the body's inner harmony.

The Plough posture can be practised from thirty seconds up to five minutes. It is of great benefit for mental concentration, especially helping those who are overtly extroverted to gain a good degree of introversion whilst at the same time calming the whole body and mind.

Apart from that it enlivens the different organs in the stomach area and helps to reduce the problem of lack of appetite, indigestion, belching

If one suffers from problems with gas, which cause acute pain in the abdomen, this posture can release the gas from the bowels and promotes a feeling of relaxation.

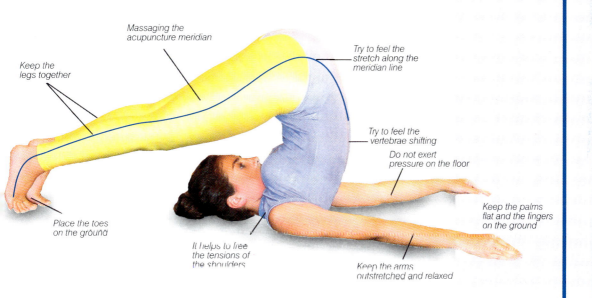

- Massaging the acupuncture meridian
- Keep the legs together
- Place the toes on the ground
- Try to feel the stretch along the meridian line
- Try to feel the vertebrae shifting
- Do not exert pressure on the floor
- It helps to free the tensions of the shoulders
- Keep the palms flat and the fingers on the ground
- Keep the arms outstretched and relaxed

CAUTION:
This ásana should be avoided by those who suffer from heart and lung disorders.

25

vrkṣāsana

In Saṁskṛta vrkśa means tree, so this is named the tree posture.

BENEFITS

This posture helps to achieve strong concentration, attaining a balance between mind and body, and leading one towards introversion.

Aids in achieving proper breathing, that is deep, steady and replenishing. While following the prescribed breathing system, the mind will become especially attentive.

It maintains a balance from head to the foot.

While reaching high like a tree the back is stretched.

While maintaining the balance in the body during this āsana, one has to stand on ones foot and as a result of that the veins of the leg become very strong.

It is not easy for everyone to stand on one leg on the floor. Therefore those who might have any difficulty in standing on one leg on the floor should stand near to a pillar or a wall for supporting the body weight in the beginning of the practice.

From a standing position place the left foot against the right inner thigh. Keep the leg straight with the right foot placed firmly on the floor. Stretch the arms above the head, palms touching. Concentrate the eyes on a fixed point keeping the body erect.

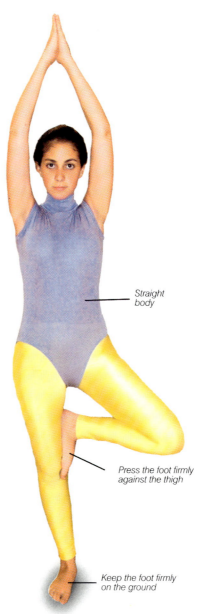

Straight body

Press the foot firmly against the thigh

Keep the foot firmly on the ground

TREE POSTURE

Palms together

Stretch the arms

Eyes are one pointed

Maintain a regular breathing system.
One round means completing the procedure in both legs.
Practise four rounds.

HOW TO DO

Stay in that position for six to eight seconds.

Keep the lifted hands light and firm. The leg on which you are standing should also be tight, firm and straight.

After staying in this position for a maximum of eight seconds, return to the position of readiness with the following process.

Slowly and rhythmically bring the lifted arms down to your side.

Continue to breath slowly and deeply.

One round means completing the procedure in both legs.

Practice four rounds.

26 granthimuktāsana

In Saṁskṛta granthi means joint and mukta means to free, to loosen.

BENEFITS

This posture is particularly beneficial for the joints and bones of the body, relieving gout and arthritis mainly in the knees and elbows.

It strengthens the nervous system and helps cleanse the body and limbs of all toxins.

Because of it's balancing nature it helps the relationship between body and mind leading one to a higher level of attentiveness.

It alleviates problems of weakness, low energy and vitality and increases the flexibility of the knees

Rejuvenates the inactive nerves in the body

Increases internal concentration. One can close the eyes and achieve even more concentration

Practising this posture with perseverance one will attain much benefit, helping to attain greater and greater peace of mind.

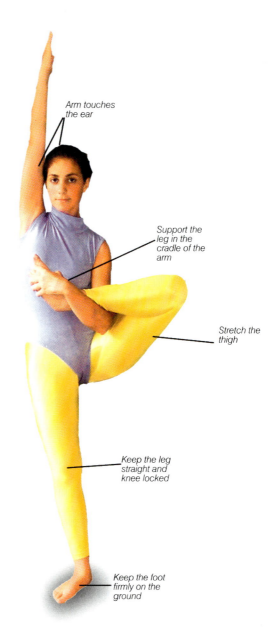

Arm touches the ear

Support the leg in the cradle of the arm

Stretch the thigh

Keep the leg straight and knee locked

Keep the foot firmly on the ground

JOINT LOOSENING POSTURE

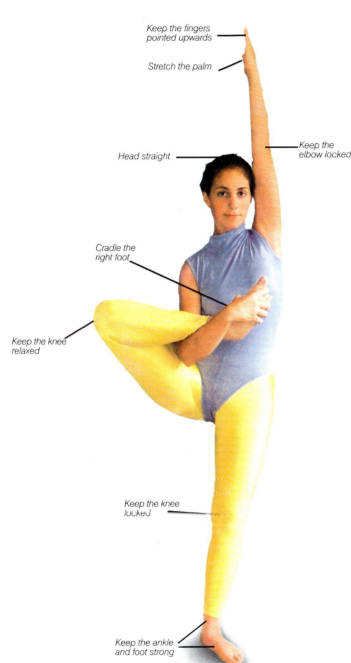

Keep the fingers pointed upwards
Stretch the palm
Keep the elbow locked
Head straight
Cradle the right foot
Keep the knee relaxed
Keep the knee locked
Keep the ankle and foot strong

HOW TO DO

In preparation for this posture one may also practise this in sitting position.

One should stand straight and take hold of the left ankle with the right hand, gradually raising the foot as high as possible.

At the same time raise the left arm above the head.

Inhale as you raise the foot then exhale and maintain this position for eight seconds.

Switch legs and repeat the process.

This makes one complete round. Practise four rounds.

NOTE:
It is better to do this posture on a carpeted floor rather than standing on a plastic mat. One can't make the body straight and firm and maintain proper balance on the soft mats, which are usually sold in stores for yoga practice.

27

BENEFITS

Body and mind are completely rested, leading to a greater degree of concentration.

It helps the body to release toxins in the back. Keeping a strong and supple spine will make one feel energetic and youthful.

It helps acquire flexibility in the back

This posture releases tiredness, leaving the body and mind refreshed

It is beneficial for the liver, pancreas, stomach and spleen.

ATTENTION:
a) One should start practicing it after being accustomed to Sarváungásana and Vipariitakaraṅi mudrá*.
b) In the beginning of starting the practice of this ásana, one should do it in the afternoon time instead of morning time

shivásana
SHIVÁSANA

Lie down on the floor, assuming the position of shoulder stand. From this upright position bend the knees and gradually lower them toward the ground placing them either side of the head.

Caution should be taken not to force this position. One should lower the knees gradually to the ground.

Hold from thirty seconds to five minutes.

This ásana is very good for flexing the back.

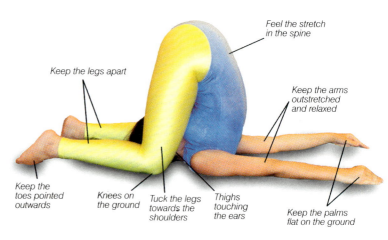

Feel the stretch in the spine
Keep the legs apart
Keep the arms outstretched and relaxed
Keep the toes pointed outwards
Knees on the ground
Tuck the legs towards the shoulders
Thighs touching the ears
Keep the palms flat on the ground

Bring the knees toward the ears and opening the thighs place the knees either side of the head. Keep the arms outstretched and pointing forwards.

Breathe slowly and deeply, keeping the body and mind as tranquil as possible.

*Reverse Posture: The differences between Vipariitakaráni Mudrá and Sarváungásana are that; in Vipariitakaráni Mudrá, the body is not straight and the mind is fixed at the tip of the nose or at the navel.

shavásana
SHAVÁSANA

Shava means corpse in Saṁskṛta. Though this posture is called corpse posture, it is an ásana for deep relaxation and rest.

STEP 1

This posture is practised at the end of the yoga routine as a deep relaxation. If you wish to attain the best results from your yoga routine you should also perform shavásana for a short time between each pose.

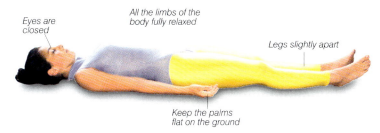

Eyes are closed
All the limbs of the body fully relaxed
Legs slightly apart
Keep the palms flat on the ground

Lie on the back with the arms outstretched to the sides, palms facing upwards, eyes closed in a perfectly relaxed position. Breathe slowly and deeply.

Some tips to aid in deeper rest. Find a quiet place which doesn't stimulate your sensory and motor organs. Put on some soft music, helping to turn the inwards. Close the eyes and focussing on your breathing relax the entire body from head to toe. Like a dead body keep absolutely still and quiet and concentrate on your breathing. Feel, your whole body is resting. Remain in this position for some time. Try to go beyond time, place and person, go beyond all the physical senses and feel the purity within. As your body relaxes yawning may come but try to maintain an awakening state.

Minimum duration for this ásana is two minutes. After Shavásana you will feel refreshed and light.

One can do it even up to 15 minutes in some special circumstances under which one is not allowed to do many other common ásanas.

28
BENEFITS

Very good for alleviating high blood pressure, heart disease and cancer type fatal diseases.

If the body is very weak it is recommended to practise this ásana above all others.

It's revitalising effects aid the mind even more than the body.

Helps one to develop the habit of deep inhalation and long exhalation.

Unleashes a subtle energy in the mind which leads to creative expression and higher emotions such as love.

The more one practises this ásana the more one gets control of the mind over body.

It readies the mind for long and deep meditation.

This posture can be done anytime as it works to refresh the practitioner giving both a physical and psychic boost.

Shavásana can be practised after the completion of each ásana leading to an increase in the effectiveness of each pose.

SOME COMMON GUIDELINES FOR NATURAL AND HEALTHY LIVING

We, the humans are at liberty to follow or to ridicule rules and regulations in our divine life. In our daily life, we must follow some natural rules, as the creator himself follows His own rule in His creation. The cause of almost all diseases is nothing but the violation of the natural system.

When we follow the rules of utilising natural sources such as water, air, earth and sunshine, we automatically become a natural human being and out of the grace of nature we maintain a good and healthy life. On the other hand, when we submit ourselves to chemical and artificial medicines, they may cure a certain problem for a year or so, but ultimately another problem will manifest itself sooner or later.

People can survive many days without food. But without drinking water people can hardly live more than a week. Air is also more essential than water. One will have a life and death problem without breathing even for a couple of minutes. So, for our survival both air and water are most important.

Our body's liquid factor is almost 70%. This watery portion of the body is lost through excretion, urine, perspiration and breathing. So, one should drink 3 to 4 litres of water daily. This will replace lost fluid and help to flush toxins and impurities out from the body.

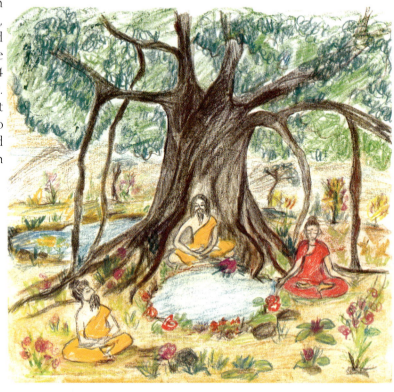

Life sparkles in an environment of earth and water getting energy from the sun and air.

The ancient yogis who lived simply in the deep forest near clean open water, under clear skies and open space and who meditated deeply with firm determination, represent the highest evolution of human beings.

EARTH

In naturopathy, the curative power of earth is second to the power of water. By applying the mud pad a lot of diseases can be cured. It has been found that in some instances mud cures more than water or hydrotherapy. Mud is used for treatment purposes by applying it to the hands, legs, head, neck and around the eyes and in some instances to the entire body.

A mudpack or earth can be used to cure diseases of the intestines, stomach, uterus and kidneys. Because the earth has such natural curative abilities, one should try to walk outdoors without shoes at times. Of course this should only be done in a clean natural environment and never on ground contaminated by city pollution.

By the way, I would like to mention that walking bare foot on the grass in the morning is also quite beneficial.

WATER, THE LIFE IN ITSELF

"Nectar of the golden life, of health and vitality."

We must choose drinking water carefully. It is better to use well water or spring water rather than tap water. Most tap water comes from surface reservoirs formed from rivers, streams and lakes. Well-water comes primarily from ground water supplies and can vary greatly in its mineral content. It is a rich source of nutritional minerals such as iron, zinc, selenium, magnesium or calcium. Unfortunately, ground water may contain toxic heavy metals or agricultural or industrial chemical pollutants such as pesticides, gasoline-by-products, etc. Spring water is the natural water found in surface or underground springs. As I am sure you are aware this water from natural springs tastes very different from other water and is a very refreshing drink

Water is the substance we need most; good drinking water is so important to health. We should know about the water we use and what it contains. If there is any water we doubt, we must get it checked. Filtration is the best way to insure that the quality of the water you drink is pure and free of contaminants. Water is essential for life and drinking the right amount of pure healthy water is important to optimum health. All the beverages we drink – tea, coffee, sodas, beer are basically water that contains other ingredients as well. Drinking good water is still the best way for obtaining our fluid requirement.

We loose water daily through our skin, urine, bowels and lungs. About half of our water losses can be replaced with the water content in the food. The remaining half requires specific fluid intake, primarily from drinking good water. Caffeinated beverages, like coffee, tea, cocoa, colas and alcoholic drinks do not contribute to the volume of water we drink because they act as diuretics in the body causing fluid loss.

It is best to consume water at various intervals during the course of the day. Drinking about one glass (eight ounce) of water every hour is optimum. It is also best to drink water an hour before or after meals but not during the meal itself. This is because water can dilute the digestive juices and reduce the digestion of our food as well as blocking the assimilation of nutrients. Drink one or two glasses ½ hour before going to bed to help flush out the system. Drinking a lot of water is also a therapy for skin diseases and constipation.

System for drinking water: Just after getting up in the morning, perform utkśepa mudrá (see page 71), and sip a small cup of water. Again after taking bath, drink another glass of water preferably with fresh lemon juice added. Water should be taken at 70° Farenheit (14° Celsius). It works like tonic for the stomach. Too cold water should not be drunk. Water should be taken in small amount many times a day.

SUNBATH

The sun is the source of all energy. The current of the water and force of the air, growth of the flora and fauna, human beings – everything depends on the big sun.

Wherever there is sunshine, there lies beauty, life and vitality. Observe the difference when vegetables are grown with plenty of sunshine and when they are not. Similarly cows, from which we get milk, produce less vitamin D when they don't enjoy grass outside and are confined inside in barns. In order to increase the vitamin levels in milk, cows needs to be free to graze more outside in open green fields.

Sunrays provide infinite benefits to the human body. They enhance the growth of white and red corpuscles, which boost the body's immune capacity. Out of this sunshine, blood-circulation increases, which is helpful for many diseases. It is also good for insomnia and lack of appetite.

With the help of sunshine, one can be cured from poor liver function, which is the cause of many diseases. Sunbathing increases mental energy. The sunrays have the capacity to kill all kinds of germs and bacteria around us.

The sunrays are a natural source of energy, available free of charge and in abundance. These have a healing power and therapeutic value by converting the inactive vitamin D in our bodies to its active form, which is essential for healthy bones.

There is a thirst for limitlessness in every human being

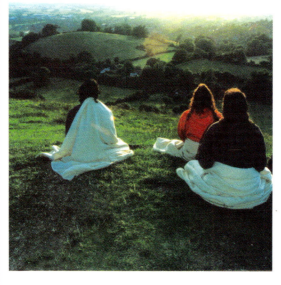

The open sky, clean air, green grass encourages the meditating yogis in Glastonbury (England) to go within in deep meditation. by taking fresh air and the soothing touch of the crimson dawn.

It is useful in correcting the deficiency or excess of a particular chemical in any part of the body.

The early rays of the sun are beneficial in activating the pituitary gland.

Solarization of water, oil or granulated sugar can be achieved by exposing these to the sun in a coloured bottle.

It produces medicinal properties in the substances.

AIR

The human respiratory system takes oxygen from the bloodstream and carries it to all the body cells, where it is used to release energy from food during aerobic respiration. Breathing also allows the expulsion of waste products such as carbon dioxide into the air.

Pure and fresh air has the power to cure diseases. Breathing in as fully as possible allows the air the opportunity to be completely absorbed by the lungs.

Yogic science explains the relationship between the air we breathe and pránáh, or vital life energy that is present in every structure or living system. This science is called Pránáyáma. It is described in more detail under the heading The Eight Steps of Self-Realisation.

AIR - BATH

If we observe nature and natural phenomena, we see that the birds and animals that roam free get fewer problems than human beings because they are exposed to the clean fresh air of nature. As a result, they look so beautiful, healthy and full of life. Similarly, the people in cosmopolitan cities suffer ill health more than the tribal and village people who are far away from the pollution of the city.

When one is confined in the house, in a city-life, one gets bad health due to poison effect of unclean air and toxins on the blood, and secondly one gets problems to maintain proper temperature in the body.

Two gateways exist where poison may enter our bodies, and these are the mouth and the nose. Just as bad food causes us to become ill, so does dirty, and polluted air. The more we breathe polluted air the more it will cause problems in our body's blood supply, making us unhealthy. As you know, when we exhale waste and poisonous gases are expelled from our bodies. For this reason sleeping with blankets covering one's face during the winter can cause poisonous carbonic acid to enter the body. This will cause the condition of the blood to deteriorate and should be avoided.

In the same way, it is also unhealthy to live in a house that is closed up tight without good ventilation. It is much healthier to breathe cool, dry fresh air with low humidity than indoor air, which may be even more polluted than the outdoor air found in large cities. If one lives in a house that does not have proper ventilation one will find that their health will deteriorate and they will lose their digestive capacity and appetite. In this deteriorated state any type of stress or tension may lead one to experience a heart attack or other cardiac problems.

To increase appetite, the best method is to walk in the free and clean air. That is called air-bath. It increases ones cognitive capacity, opens the mind and removes stress and tension. It helps the thyroid and adrenal glands. It is also beneficial for the skin.

As I have mentioned before, one can stay without water hardly a week or so. But without air life gets suffocated. So, one must know how to utilise this precious wealth in our life. In yoga techniques the fourth state is pránáyáma, which deals with the breathing technique. In relaxation, one is supposed to take free slow, smooth and continual breathing. We know the last breath signals an end in our life. So, in life, when we are capable to breath, we should do it with all feeling and system.

The Vegetarian Pyramid

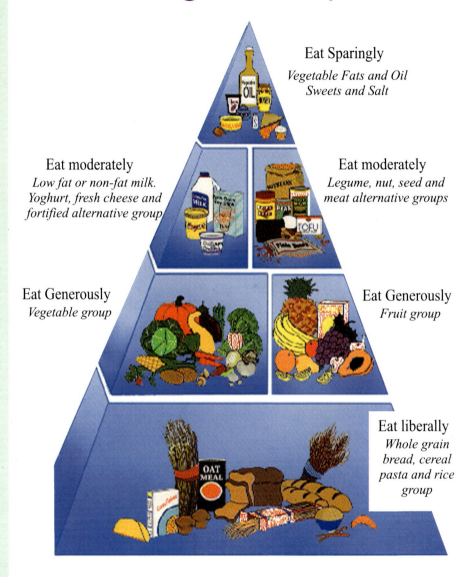

Eat Sparingly
*Vegetable Fats and Oil
Sweets and Salt*

Eat moderately
*Low fat or non-fat milk.
Yoghurt, fresh cheese and
fortified alternative group*

Eat moderately
*Legume, nut, seed and
meat alternative groups*

Eat Generously
Vegetable group

Eat Generously
Fruit group

Eat liberally
*Whole grain
bread, cereal
pasta and rice
group*

One can stay healthy with sound mind body and spirit through the entire life time. By making the decision to eat food that is good for us physically, mentally and spiritually (sentient food), we are empowered, because we are choosing a healthy lifestyle, now and for our future.

FOOD

It has always been said that "We are what we eat" and that having a sound healthy body depends on our taking proper amounts of nutritious foods. We should only eat that food which is helpful in keeping the body and mind sentient. According to Yoga philosophy, each object or entity in the universe possesses in different proportions, the characteristics of these three forces (guńas). These forces are known as sentient, mutative, and static. The sentient force is a force of evolution, the mutative force is a force of change, and the static force is a force of degradation. They influence the whole creation, which is, in all its parts, dominated by one or the other principle – and food is no exception.

Sentient (sáttvik) food: Food that produces sentient cells and is thus good for both physical and mental growth is sentient. Examples of sentient food are rice, wheat, all kinds of beans, fruits, milk and milk products and most of the green vegetables.

Mutative (rájasik) food: Food that is good for the body but may or may not be good for the mind – but is certainly not harmful – is considered mutative. Foods that do not fall into the sentient or static categories are of mutative or rájasik nature. Small amounts of tea, cocoa and similar stimulant drinks, certain varieties of spices are in the mutative category.

Static (támasik) food: Food that is harmful for the mind and may or may not be good for the body is static. These foods include onion, garlic, wine, stale and rotten food, meat of most of the animals, fish, eggs, etc.

Our physical and mental development depends on our food. The physical body of human being is nothing but a composed form of countless cells. Each of these cells has its individual mind. Cells generously grow out of light, air, water and the nutrients derived from what we eat. The nature of food and drink therefore, has a definite effect upon the cells, and also influences the mind.

The human being is dominated mainly by the mind. Life is more a psychic experience than a physical one. It is the mind that decides to do good things and bad acts. In order to do spiritual practice one needs a calm, quiet and concentrated mind and for that sentient food is indispensable. If someone is agitated by the instincts or vrttis, the mind will not be relaxed and it will be difficult to lead the mind to higher pursuits. So those who want to lead a simple, synthetic spiritual life must control the food intake, so that he/she can practice meditation, concentration and contemplation properly. It is said,

"Áhárashuddhao Sattvashuddhih."

"A sentient diet produces a sentient body with sentient mind."

REFLEXOLOGY

Our entire body is intertwined with the nervous system, which binds each and every organ, glands and other structures. The foot is one of the ending points of the nerves. So, foot reflexology is based on the reflex point on the feet that correspond to the different organs of the body. Reflexology is a method of massaging the reflex point and stimulating the area corresponding to the affected part of the body to cause positive reactions and relaxation.

The history of reflexology goes back to 5000 years ago, when the technique of acupuncture started in India and China. Related documents were discovered in Egypt 2500-2300 BC.

In our modern age Dr. William H. Fitzgerald, an American physician discovered 'Zone Therapy'. All organs, glands and the entire nervous system fall into ten zones. The Zone theory can be told as the origin of reflexology. It is a common assumption that the hands and feet are the main areas to which the techniques of reflexology can be applied very effectively.

Science tells us that the body is an electro-magnetic field. One becomes ill or diseased when the balance of the electromagnetic field of the body is not in equilibrium; in this condition the glands too will be affected. When you apply pressure over the appropriate nerve-endings, the crystalline deposits are pulverized, and as a result of this, the electro-magnetic currents start to flow freely again and one gets relaxed.

The benefit of reflexology is that it relaxes the inner organs. By reducing tension it cures a lot of diseases, which are originated from the stress and strain. In reflexology, the foot is the mirror of the body-mind. It reflects the blockages when the body gets upset and it looses the equilibrium. Because of the bad habits, the body piles up a lot of harmful deposits around the terminal nerve endings. This physical obstruction of that zone causes blockages with toxin poisoning which creates diseases related to liver, calcification, gouts, arthritis, kidney problems, diseases of the blood circulatory system, nervous diseases and many others. So the easy and practical cure for all the diseases is the regular practice of reflexology. Toxins must be removed from the body through the nerve endings of the feet. Without taking help from others, one can help even oneself. One has to know the pressure points from some experienced teacher and apply it in everyday life.

You touch your own body; feel loved and valued by your own being. Softly exert pressure on yourself and it will help. You will keep pace with the pressure of poisoned society. You can develop feeling your own body and mind with proper sensation and can share the language of touch with the feeling of love, youthfulness and service.

Develop your healing powers, remove stress and tension.!

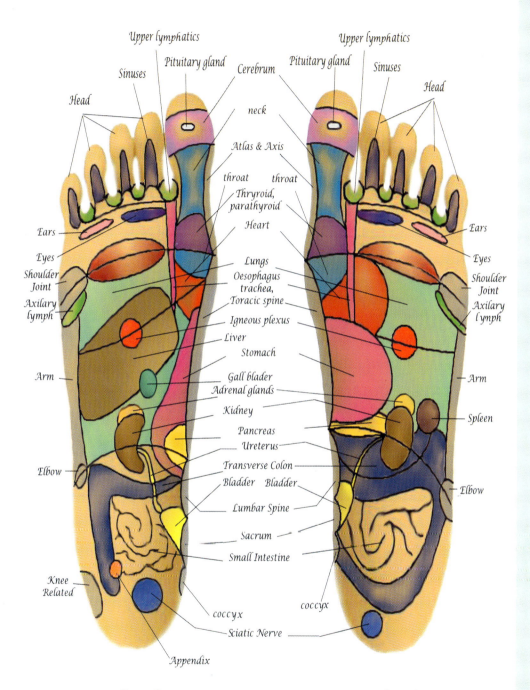

THE SYSTEM FOR PRACTICING YOGA ÁSANAS

For those who want to get maximum benefit from ásanas, one should try to follow the following rules:

• After one gets up in the morning, clean the bowels; take bath; then start Yoga ásanas. The bath has four different effects on body and mind

1- It makes one feel light and relaxed;
2- It transforms the static energy of the body to the subtle energy of body-mind
3- It brings vitality in life, from which comes a feeling of happiness;
4- It helps to perform ásanas and meditation more easily. In case you want to take bath after ásanas, it should not be taken with cool water.

• If you want to perform ásanas in the evening time, it is better to do it before the evening meal.

• There should be silence in the room. Use a blanket folded several times or a yoga mat.

• While doing ásanas one should wear clothes appropriate for the temperature of the room. If one feels that the temperature is comfortable, one can use the minimum clothes, i.e. just underwear.

• While doing ásanas one should not speak. In this way, this energy is channelized inwards bringing the maximum benefit.

• Try to notice the breathing and keep it systematic while performing the ásanas

• Gradually proceed to the ásanas you want to do, keeping in mind the ideation and feeling of the benefits for each posture while performing them

• You can begin ásanas by relaxing in Shavásana posture.

• We are doing ásanas to overcome temperamental behaviour; before you begin try to be in a calm, quiet and gentle mood.

• One will get the benefit of each ásana gradually. One should patiently proceed with the practice of ásanas.

• Yoga is a practical science, so one should try to learn it from an experienced person.

• Wholesome meals make one feel light. So one should take substantial food. To take a complete meal does not mean to fill up the stomach.

• While suffering from a cold or fever, one should not do ásanas.

• While doing ásanas, one should not force oneself. Rather, take a gradual approach and follow the guidance of the teacher.

- Between each change of posture, it is preferable to lay down in shavásana for approximately one minute. During this time one should ideate on and feel the benefit of the ásana just completed.

- To do ásanas does not mean to become tired or fatigued. While practicing, one should try to find oneself relaxed, free and introverted.

- To get the best benefit of ásanas, one should try to practice twice a day. If you cannot do it twice a day, it should be once, preferably in the morning, on an empty stomach.

- Never practise ásanas with a full stomach. After taking a heavy meal, there should be at least a 3-hour gap.

- After ásanas are finished, one should not come into contact with water for 20 minutes. Also one should not drink water for at least 10 minutes.

- At the end of ásanas, one should do self-massage and relax in shavásana.

- Ásanas should never be done in a poorly ventilated room, such as basements, but while performing it there should be no air current or wind in direct contact with the body.

- Do not perform ásanas during menstruation. At that time practise massage and shavásana.

- Nails should be kept short. Watch, rings, ornaments etc. should not be worn.

- One can start ásanas after 12 years of age. Yet there are some prescribed postures for children, which may be done under the guidance of an experienced practitioner. According to different ages the most beneficial ásanas also change.

- The series of ásanas have a proper order. If one does not find out how to arrange them, it is better to do easier ásanas followed by more difficult ones.

- For women and men there are some different basic ásanas.

- If someone wants to do sports or other exercise, it should be done before ásanas. Walking is suitable after ásanas

- Those who perform regular meditation, should do ásanas after meditation.

- It is preferable to perform ásanas at a fixed time everyday to obtain maximum benefits.

- One should learn ásanas from an experienced teacher. For the first six months of practice, one should get the guidance of a competent instructor.

- While dong ásanas, breathing should always be through the nose.

- It is better not to perform ásanas immediately after bath.

- Whatever time or age one begins doing ásanas, to get the real benefits, one has to be very diligent, respectful and have complete mental acceptance of the system. In this way, one will certainly get the benefit in three to four months.

- If suffering from chronic disease, then one must practice systematically for one year to achieve the benefits.

- Do ásanas everyday. Practice should only be missed at the time of some particular disease. Ásanas should be practiced in a systematic and habitual way. It should be done as a duty with feeling.

- In the beginning it may be difficult to make the habit, but after it will become as habitualized as brushing the teeth, or taking a bath.

- If performed regularly, seven to eight ásanas are enough for a day.

- For those with intolerable physical pain or severe headache (migraine), three to four ásanas per day is enough.

- Those who have health problems such as hypertension, blood pressure, heart problems, lung complications, slip disc, rheumatism, ulcer, persistent indigestion, constipation should not take any steps without seeking the advice of a professional instructor.

- During pregnancy practicing ásanas up to the first three months is okay. There after only practice as per the instruction of an experienced teacher.

- For practicing ásanas there is no diet prescription. Simply one should have balanced, substantial and vegetarian diet for getting maximum benefit from the practice.

- Through the perfect practice of ásanas, one will feel lightness in the body and bliss in the mind. One should try to keep those feelings by performing ásanas as precisely as possible.

- Try to do ásanas with a deep mind and inner feeling like a meditation. In this way many positive things will happen in life.

ANTI- AGING: THE LONGEVITY PROGRAM

Some important factors that stop increase aging and degeneration are mentioned here:

• Sentient food, fresh air, positive thinking, constructive selfless work, proper conduct and behaviour.

• Get up, perform utks'epa múdra, attend to the call of nature and devote some time in remembering the Cosmic Consciousness.

• Morning walk with proper breathing

• Take bath, perform ásanas and meditation and get ready to perform your routine jobs.

• The most correct and proper way to take bath is to pour water on the navel area, then drop water from top of your body down the back from the pineal gland.

• If you don't take a full bath, take a half-bath. The system is: keeping water in the mouth and splash the eyes, spitting out the water afterwards. This also helps one to have clear vision. Wash the genital area, arms from elbows down, legs from knees down. The same thing should be done before and after food and sleep.

• Lemon water with salt, fruit juice, fruit and cereals are good in the morning. At noon-time, soup, leafy and green vegetables and curd water is beneficial. At night time milk is more helpful.

• At least 3 to 4 litres of water should be taken each day.

• There should be a gap of 3 to 4 hours between meals. Stomach-full eating habit is harmful for the body.

• While eating, silence is better. Instead of talking, one should concentrate in chewing many times.

• Manual labour is good all the time. If there is no scope, yoga ásanas should be done compulsorily.

• Cultivating fine arts is creative and good for mind. Instead of gossiping, mudslinging and unhealthy criticism, it is better to utilize the time for social service and personal physico-psycho-spiritual development.

•We should remember. 'Early to bed, early to rise...

• After dinner one should walk and go to bed afterwards. One should finish eating before 9pm.

• Day-sleep and night awakening is bad for health.

• Fasting at least twice a month.

• Proper time for food, sleep, study, work, recreation, meditation and exercise is the secret of longevity.

ÁSANAS IN STANDING POSITION

ÁSANAS TABLE

BHÁVÁSANA

PADAHASTÁSANA

KARMÁSANA - I

KARMÁSANA - II

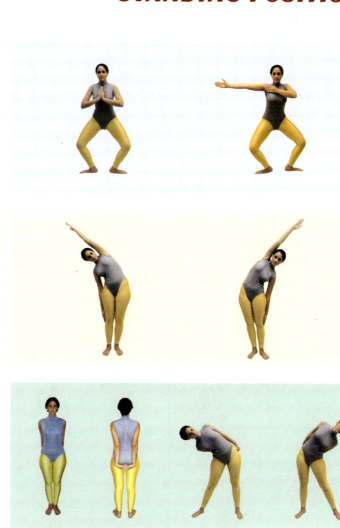

GOOD FOR THE SPINE

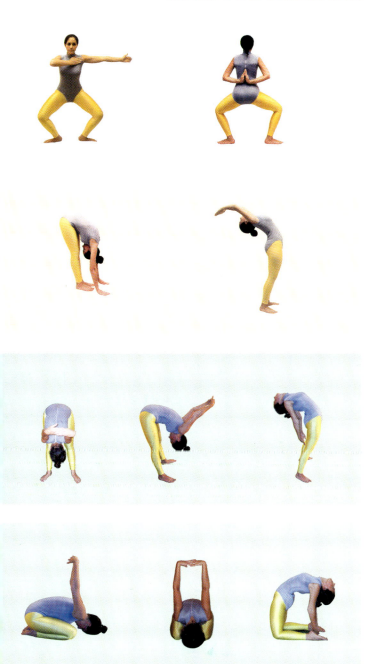

Helps to keep the spine straight; one develops the habit of standing erect. The muscles of the knees become strong. Breathing should be free, natural and slow. All four positions make one round. Each round should be done four times.

While doing this ásana, the hands and the arms should be together, with the arms touching the ears. While going down one should exhale. While coming up, one should inhale. In each position, one should wait for 8 seconds. 4 positions make one round. It should be done for 4 rounds.

One becomes energetic and active, therefore the name of this posture is karmásana. If someone is lethargic, one can remove this lethargy by practicing this posture daily. The hands are clenched, fingers interlocked, knees kept straight. The breathing system should be followed. Do 4 rounds.

CAUTION
Forcing oneself while bending backward and forward should not be done by those having high blood pressure.

ÁSANAS TABLE

ÁSANAS IN STANDING POSITION

VIIRA BHADRÁSAN

PÁRŚVOTTANÁSAN

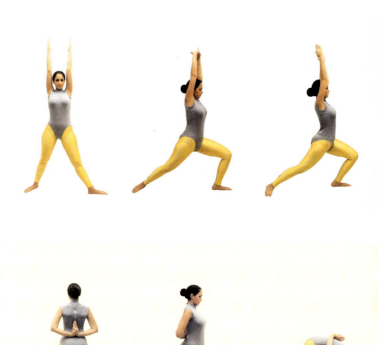

PÁRŚVOTTANÁSAN

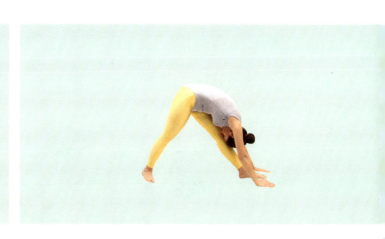

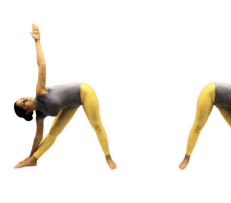

TRIKONÁSAN

"Triangular posture". The body should be kept erect. The knees should be straight. Arms should be perpendicular to the floor. Breathing is free and natural.

Each position should be done for 4 rounds.

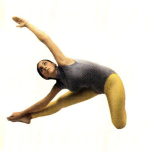
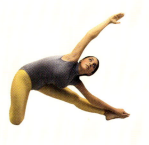

PARIGHÁSANA

Stand erect and keep the body in proper position.

It makes the whole body flexible.

It creates self-confidence and gives fighting spirit.

The knees are made strong.

It is good for removing the pain of hips and lower back.

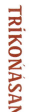

PRASÁRITA PADOTTANÁSANA

CAUTION!
The postures that make one bend are not suitable for those who are pregnant.

ÁSANAS TABLE

ÁSANAS IN STANDING POSITION

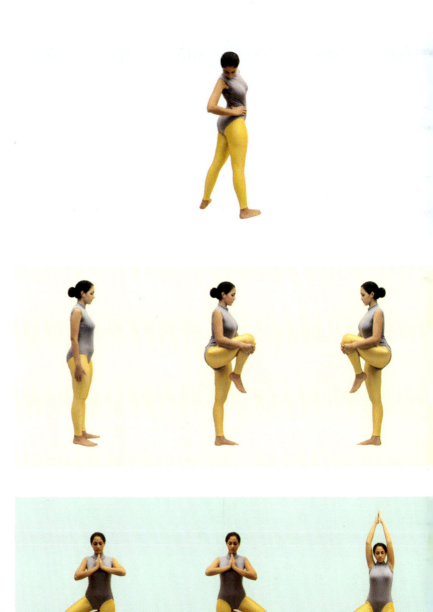

BALANCE POSTURES

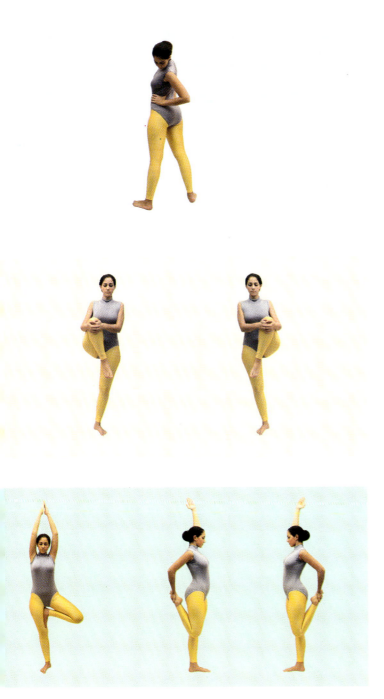

Keep the body erect; hold the waist, turn to the right looking at the heel of the left leg. The breathing system is natural, not regulated.
One trip is: one left turn and one right turn.
Repeat 4 trips.
Develops the neck, waist and lumbar regions of the spine. It is also helpful for stiff cramp in neck or back. These are the positions that prepare one in the gradual process towards developing balance and concentration.

The right and left legs are pressed towards the stomach. This strengthens the muscles of both legs and stomach. Try to do this ásana with concentration and free breathing.

These are the balance postures.
In the beginning, one should do with open eyes fixed at one point. Gradually one can do it closing the eyes.
It will help in concentration.

The breathing is free. Each trip can be done four times.

ÁSANAS TABLE

ÁSANAS IN SITTING POSITION

BADDHA KOŃÁSAN

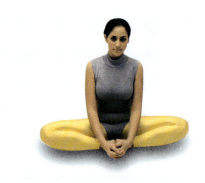

UPAVÍŚTA KOŃÁSAN

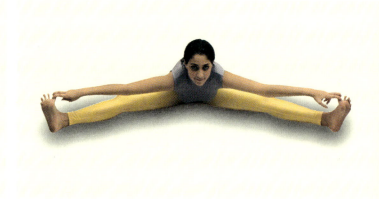

UTKAŤA KÚRMAKÁSANA

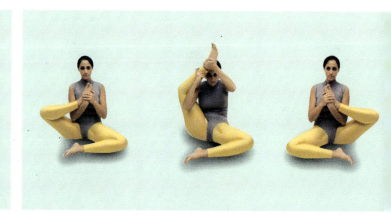

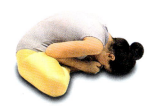

In the beginning one should sit straight; then, holding the feet, gradually bend down while exhaling. One can concentrate the mind on the third eye cakra. Try to touch the forehead with the toes.

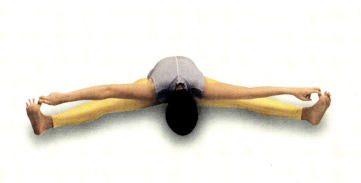

This is the triangle posture in sitting position. It makes the knees and all the vertebrae of the spine flexible. While going down, breathe out; while going up, breathe in, holding the breath in that posture for eight seconds. Do four repetitions.

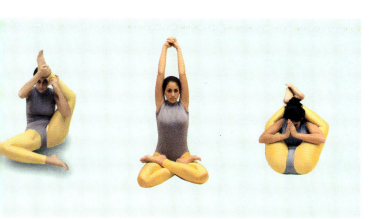

The first two postures prepare for this ásana. They help to make all the joints of the leg flexible.
First try to bring the foot towards the stomach, and upwards. Finally, when one can lift, the other foot can follow interlocking behind the head. By doing this ásana one can get the benefit as if doing many ásanas.

ÁSANAS TABLE

ÁSANAS ON THE FLOOR

Develops balance strenghtens the legs.

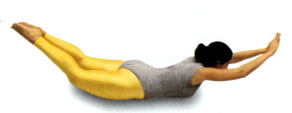

The internal organs develop strength and resilience through these postures.

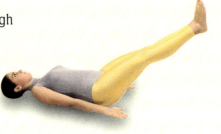

The legs should be at 30° from the floor.

The postures here are the preparation for doing "hand stand" or "shoulder stand". Performing these, one will gradually strengthen the back.

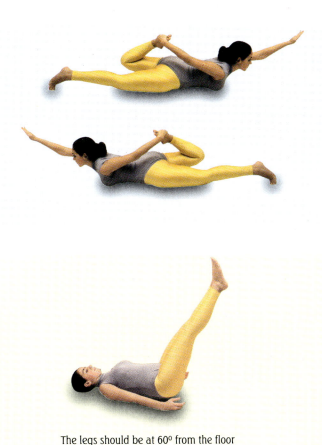

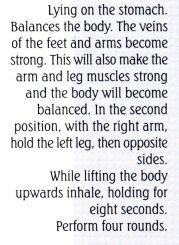

Lying on the stomach. Balances the body. The veins of the feet and arms become strong. This will also make the arm and leg muscles strong and the body will become balanced. In the second position, with the right arm, hold the left leg, then opposite sides.
While lifting the body upwards inhale, holding for eight seconds.
Perform four rounds.

Camel Posture
It activates the muscles around the stomach, intestine and liver. The organs of this region are all benefited by this posture. It also massages the spine.

Keep the legs at 30º and 60º from the floor, with no time limit.

The legs should be at 60º from the floor

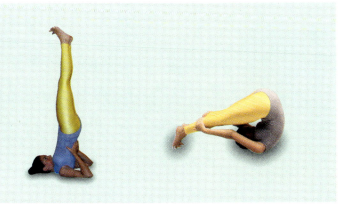

By doing these ásanas one can be cured of the diseases related to the neck, spine and coccyx.

The average time for staying in the position is three minutes.
It can be done 3 or 4 times.

Saṁskṛta Glossary

We have used Roman Saṁskṛta (Sanskrit) alphabet. It helps the readers to pronounce the words correctly.

Ácárya	Teacher for spiritual meditation.
Aham	I do, part of the mind.
Ánanda	Cosmic bliss; transcendental happiness experienced when the individual mind merges in Cosmic being.
Ánanda Márga	Path of Bliss; (ananda=bliss; marga=path); the spiritual practices and ideology of Shrii Shrii Ánandamúrti; the organization formed by Shrii Shrii Ánandamúrti
Ásana	lit. posture comfortably held; physical posture of yoga.
Aśtáuṅga	Eight limbs.
Átma, átman	The individual, individual spirit.
Áyúrveda	Science of life and death, Indian natural way of medicine.
Bhakti	Spiritual devotion; love for the Supreme.
Bhakti yoga	Yoga of devotion.
Bháva	Ideation.
Bhuta	Living beings.
Biija	A seed, source, origin, beginning.
Brahma	Supreme Consciousness.
Cakra	Psychic energy center.
Cintá	Disturbed thought, anxious thought.
Citta	Mind stuff or ectoplasm; the part of the mind which takes the shape of sensory data or physical actions.
Dháraṅá	Concentration on a fixed point
Dharma	Characteristic, property.
Dhyána	lit. flowing of the mind; meditation; a pure state of absorption in the Supreme.
Guru	lit. gu= darkness; ru=light; the preceptor who removes ignorance with light and gives light.
Iśta	Goal.
Iidá	A channel of psychic energy in the body corresponding to the sympathetic nervous system.
Jinána	Spiritual knowledge, wisdom.
Karma	An act; universal law of cause and effect.
Kośa	lit. sheath; layer of the mind.
Kula Kuṅdalinii	lit. coiled serpentine force; psycho-spiritual energy dormant in the base of the spine.
Mantra	lit. which liberates the mind; a sound vibration used to focus on meditation incantation.
Mudrá	A practice of hatha yoga.
Muni	Saint.
Náma	Name.
Nádi	A psychic energy channel in the body.
Pátainjali	Propounder or systematizer of Aśtáuṅga Yoga
Piuṅgalá	Energy channel ending at the right nostril.
Prakrti	Operative Principle of Brahma; the binding force.
Práṅa(h)	Vital energy, breath.
Pratyáhára	Withdrawal of senses into the mind
Puruśa	Aspect of Brahma which is Consciousness itself.
Rájá	King.
Rájádhirája	King of kings, emperor
Rśi	Sage
Rúpa	Shape an outward appearance.
Sádhaka	A spiritual aspirant.
Sádhaná	Spiritual practices; continuous effort to attain the goal.
Saṁskára	Reactive momenta; seeds of past actions in potential form.
Suśumṅá	Central channel of psychic energy within the spine.
Sútra	Aphorism.
Tantra	Which liberates from darkness and bondages.
Upaniśad	lit. upa=near; ni=down; sat=to sit sitting down near Guru to receive spiritual instructions.
Veda	Ancient knowledge
Vrtti	Propensity, mental tendency.
Yoga	lit. union; merging individual consciousness in Supreme Consciousness.
Yogi	Yoga practitioner.